Gender Madn(

M000014979

Essays from the Struggle for Dignity

Text Revision

Pre-publication Reviews and Comments:

There is no one who has written more thoughtfully than Kelley Winters about the damage inflicted on transsexual and transgender people by pseudo-scientific psychiatric nomenclature and professional arrogance. In this book, she lucidly lays out the conflicts and some potential solutions for resolving the power struggle between some psychiatrists and psychologists, who are supposedly objective authorities, and trans people themselves, who are seeking autonomy, dignity and integrity. In the battle over DSM-V, this book provides some desperately needed understanding.

Jamison Green, MFA, author of
Becoming a Visible Man

As long as our identities are regarded as a disorder we will never attain equality. Our rights and our lives depend on overturning this misogynistic idea. Kelley has been fighting for years to undo the damage this slanderous and dehumanizing diagnosis has caused.

Denise Leclair, Executive Director, International Foundation for Gender Education. See www.ifge.org

Kelley Winters has compiled a remarkable collection of short essays examining the diagnosis of Gender Identity Disorder [GID] in the DSM and the role it has played in creating mental health problems for transgender people. Dr. Winters has long been a leader in deconstructing the psychiatric labeling of people with atypical gender expressions and this book brings the discussion up-to-date.

Gender Madness in American Psychiatry examines a broad array of issues from how the GID diagnosis is used to justify reparative therapy for gender-variant children and the historical context for psychiatrically labeling of sexual minorities. Most importantly, Dr. Winters outlines the damage caused to transgender, transsexual, and other gender nonconforming people who are labeled with a mental illness. She challenges the APA committee to address ten specific issues with the GID diagnosis, a challenge that will not be easy to ignore. Gender Madness in American Psychiatry is a well-written, well-reasoned argument for the reform of Gender Identity diagnoses in the psychiatric nomenclature.

Arlene Istar Lev LCSW, CASAC, author of
Transgender Emergence and
The Complete Lesbian and Gay Parenting Guide.
See http://professionals.gidreform.org/aboutus.html

Gender Madness
in American Psychiatry

*Essays from the
Struggle for Dignity*

Text Revision

Kelley Winters, Ph.D.

With a foreword by Dan Karasic, M.D.

GID Reform Advocates
www.gidreform.org

Gender Madness in American Psychiatry
Essays from the Struggle for Dignity

Text Revision

Cover graphics by Kelley Winters.

Published by GID Reform Advocates, Dillon, Colorado
www.gidreform.org

november

Publisher Cataloging-in-Publication Data

Gender Madness in American Psychiatry: Essays from the Struggle for Dignity / Kelley Winters
        p. cm.
    Includes bibliographical references and index.
    ISBN-10: 1-4392-2388-2
    ISBN-13: 9781439223888
    1. Gender Identity Disorders.
RC560.G45 W56
616.85/83
                            2008912210

Dedication

To my sons,
who give me hope for a better world.

Never doubt that you can make a difference.

Acknowledgements

I am deeply indebted to the pioneers of gender policy reform in the *Diagnostic and Statistical Manual of Mental Disorders*, who first voiced concern about the classification of gender difference as mental illness in the 1990s and earlier: organizers of Transgender Nation, Transsexual Menace, International Conference on Transgender Law and Employment Policy, National Center for Lesbian Rights, Hermaphrodites with Attitude, National Coalition for GID Reform, Psychiatrists and Other Physicians for GID Reform and to the National Gay and Lesbian Task Force for advocacy in those early years. Frank Kameny blazed the trail in the struggle to remove homosexuality from the DSM in the 1970s and 80s, and I thank him for the vision and encouragement he shared with me.

I want to express my appreciation of those mental health care providers who are supportive and affirming of their transitioning clients. Their courage and compassion in defying derogatory psychiatric stereotypes and policies save lives and free souls.

I could not have begun this work without Sean Gardner, whose tutorage in queer literature and the English language in the Palouse Hills gave me a voice; Barbara Hammond, who helped me find my way and took a chance to coauthor a peer-reviewed presentation in feminist psychology with an engineer; and Dan Karasic, who opened doors of opportunity and insight for more than a decade.

I thank all the thoughtful people who have patiently counseled, advised, debated, inspired, encouraged and challenged me on these issues over many years: Jamison Green, Moonhawk River Stone, Dylan Scholinski, Lynn Conway, Dana Beyer, Andrea James, Arlene Lev, Holly, Randall Ehrbar, Mary Ann Horton, BJ Kamigaki, Michael-Deborah Gray, Pauline Park, Diana Cicotello, Riki Wilchins, and many others.

My special thanks go to Katie Raymond, Lisa Gilinger, Just Evelyn, Arlene Lev and readers of the GID Reform Advocates web site for reviewing these essays and providing invaluable feedback. I also thank Drs. Becky Allison, Gary Alter and Marci Bowers for input and information on surgical procedures and common health coverage practice.

I am especially grateful to the individuals and organizations who have lent their voices as advocates for GID reform. GID Reform Advocates (www.gidreform.org) are medical and mental health professionals, caregivers, scholars, researchers, students, human rights advocates, and members of the transgender, bisexual, lesbian and gay communities and their allies who advocate reform of the psychiatric classification of gender diversity as mental disorder. They represent diverse opinions on reform strategies. At the time of writing, the following are listed on the GID Reform Advocates web site:

Laura Acevedo; Ana Adelstein, Ph.D.; Margo Victoria Allen; Rebecca Allison, MD, FACC, FACP; MJ Anderson; Rachel Anderson; Renee Baker, Ph.D., LMT; Nerissa Belcher; Elizabeth Bethea, M.S.W., Ph.D.; Graham N. de Bever; Elizabeth Bhulem; Marci L. Bowers, M.D.; Cristin Brew; Andrea Brown; Gene Bujold; Sarah Burgamy; Angie Canelli, MA; Gerri Cannon; Leigha Emma Cohen; Susan G. Clark, Ph.D.; Anna Conway; Lynn Conway, Professor Emerita; Arianna Davis, Ph.D.; Madeline B. Deutsch, MD; Denise "Dee Dee" Devereaux; Lore M. Dickey, M.A.; Mara Drummond; Sidney W. Ecker, M.D., F.A.C.S.; Erica Essary; Sarah Fox, Ph.D.; Michelle Gagnon; Lisa C. Gilinger; Jamison Green, M.F.A.; Sally Goldner; Dean H Hamer, Ph.D.; Terry Lee

Harrington, R.N., N.P.; Lisa M. Hartley, ACSW-DCSW; Mikayla Howden; Laura Hurn ; Joe Ippolito, L.C.S.W; Andrea James; Olivia Jensen, Ph.D.; Ilene Jones; Matt Kailey; Dan Karasic, M.D.; Scott Kerlin, Ph.D.; Dana Beyer, M.D.; Heidi Marie Kirsch; Peter Klevius; Arlene Istar Lev, LCSW, CASAC; Savannah Nicole Logsdon; Patricia Susan Martin; Lisa Maurel, MFT; Deirdre McCloskey, Ph.D.; Jodie R. Miller; Sheila Mink; Rev. Linda Miskimen Ph.D.; Nancy L. Morgan, M.S., Ph.D.; Michele O'Mara, LCSW; Annalise Ophelian, MA; Pauline Park, Ph.D.; Sally Payne; Trey Polesky, B.S.; Stella Purvis; Kathrin Raymond, B.S.; Dr. Pega Ren; Kate Richmond, PhD; Susan P. Robbins, Ph.D., LCSW, LCDC; Michael Rogers, M.A.; Kim Schicklang; Sarah Marie Schmidt; Dylan Scholinski; Julia Serano, Ph.D.; Alexus Sheppard, B.S.E., D.D.S., F.A.G.D.; Ms. Stephanie Shockley; Gwen Smith; Debra Soshoux; Jennifer Souder; Ingrid Swenson, MSW; Wynelle Snow, M.D.; Renee Michelle Thomas, RA, IESNA; Steve Toby; Anne Vitale, Ph.D.; Rachael Wallbank; Lisa Wilson; Miriam Stone Wilson, MSW, MA; Sachi Wilson; Madeline H. Wyndzen, Ph. D.; Jessica Xavier; Teo Yother; Associated Youth Services of Peel; Fundación para la Identidad de Género (Foundation for Gender Identity); Gender Dysphoria Organization; Gender Identity Center of Colorado, Inc.; GenderPAC; Lifelines Rhode Island; Organisation Intersex International; Queers United; TransgenderASIA; and TransYouth Family Allies.

Table of Contents

Foreword

It's been over a decade since I became familiar with Kelley Winters' work towards reform of the Gender Identity Disorder diagnosis in the DSM. Dr. Winters sent me her paper, "The Disparate Classification of Gender and Sexual Orientation in American Psychiatry," and I asked her to present it as part of a session on transgender issues at the 1998 Annual Meeting of the American Psychiatric Association, in Toronto.

The 1998 APA meeting featured a session marking the 25th anniversary of the removal of the diagnosis of homosexuality from the DSM. Dr. Winters and I missed that session, since it overlapped with our own. While the APA was looking back on 25 years of progress since the 1973 decision, Dr. Winters laid out the work that remained in addressing concerns about the DSM diagnoses applied to trans people.

Like Dr. Winters, I was affected profoundly by meeting LGBT rights pioneers Frank Kameny and Barbara Gittings, and by knowing John Fryer, MD. In 2006, I had the honor of presenting Kameny and Gittings with the American Psychiatric Association's first John E. Fryer, M.D. Award, for contributions to LGBT mental health. Kameny and Gittings fought for equality for gay and lesbian people at a time when homosexuality was considered criminal behavior, socially subversive, and mental illness. They recognized that the DSM diagnosis of homosexuality reflected the prevailing societal view on homosexuality, but lacked scientific basis. The confluence of the changing views on homosexuality post-Stonewall, and the APA's desire to increase the scientific basis of the DSM helped set the stage for the removal of homosexuality from the DSM, but the change would not have happened with fearless leadership of activists outside the APA, like Kameny and Gittings, as well as those within, like Fryer, who disguised as "Dr. Anonymous" to protect his career, spoke of his experience as a gay psychiatrist at the 1972 APA Annual Meeting. The actions of these individuals were catalysts to make change happen faster than it would have otherwise.

Over the past decade, trans people have become more visible in society and more vocal in their demand for equality. During this time, Dr. Winters has worked to become one of the most prominent critics of the current Gender Identity Disorder diagnoses. She provides a rationale and a path towards diagnostic reform that could advance both mental health care and civil rights for trans people. As the APA works again to improve the scientific basis of the DSM, it remains unclear whether the conditions are right for meaningful GID reform. If change does happen, there is no doubt that Dr. Winters' thoughtful reasoning and tireless activism will be one of the catalysts for that change.

Dan Karasic, M.D.
Clinical Professor of Psychiatry
University of California, San Francisco

Introduction

At the 1971 Annual Meeting of the American Psychiatric Association, Dr. Frank Kameny, an astronomer and WWII combat veteran, took the stage and seized the microphone to denounce the classification of gay and lesbian people as mentally ill. It was the height of the Vietnam war and civil unrest. Attorney General Ramsey Clark was the keynote speaker for the APA convention at the Shoreham Hotel in Washington DC, and antiwar and gay activists were both collaborating and competing to protest the event. A pioneer of the fledgling gay rights movement, Kameny had attempted in prior years to discuss the category of homosexuality in the *Diagnostic and Statistical Manual of Mental Disorders* (DSM) with the APA leadership. They refused, insisting that "it is not in the best interests of the APA to meet with you." [1]

At a planned time in the APA's convocation ceremony, antiwar and gay rights protestors burst into the auditorium and attempted to take the stage but remarkably were fought back by elderly psychiatrists. In the mayhem, Dr. Kameny climbed the stage and told the moderator, "I'm seizing the microphone from you." The moderator responded, "Well, tell me your name and I'll introduce you." [2]

Kameny's impromptu speech to the APA that day marked an inflection point in the history of gay and lesbian civil rights.

1

This act of civil disobedience foreshadowed discussion in American psychiatry on the lack of scientific merit to the classification of homosexuality as mental illness. The subsequent removal of homosexuality from the DSM in 1973 through 1987 was instrumental in mitigating false stereotypes of mental illness and sexual deviance for gay and lesbian individuals and in enabling further gains in civil justice.[3]

More than three decades after the American Psychiatric Association voted to remove the classification of homosexuality as a mental disorder, people who do not conform to their assigned birth sex, either by inner identity or outer social expression, remain diagnosed as mentally ill in the Fourth Edition, Text Revision of the *Diagnostic and Statistical Manual of Mental Disorders* (DSM-IV-TR).[4] Published by the American Psychiatric Association, the DSM is regarded as the medical and social definition of mental disorder throughout the U.S. and Canada. It strongly influences international psychiatric nomenclature in the *International Statistical Classification of Diseases and Related Health Problems* (ICD), published by the World Health Organization.

The diagnostic categories of Gender Identity Disorder (GID) and Transvestic Fetishism (TF) in the DSM continue to raise questions of consistency, scientific validity, and human dignity. Recent revisions of the manual have made these diagnoses increasingly ambiguous and over-inclusive of false-positive diagnosis of mental illness. GID, implying "disordered" gender identity, currently implicates a broad array of gender-variant or transcendent adults, adolescents and children, who may or may not be transsexual, may or may not ever require medical transition procedures, and may or may not meet any scientific definition of mental disorder. The diagnostic category of Transvestic Fetishism (TF) labels cross-dressing by heterosexual males as a paraphilia or sexual deviance, devaluing

2

expression of femininity. These labels reinforce social stigma of madness and perversion for all gender-variant people with consequences very similar to those described by Dr. Kameny and Barbara Gittings for lesbian and gay people in the 1970s:

> "(1) To support and buttress the prejudices of society and to assist the bigots in the perpetration and perpetuation of their bigotry; and, at least equally important (2) To destroy the homosexual's self-confidence and self-esteem, impair his or her self-image, degrade his or her basic human dignity."[5]

Much like gay, lesbian and bisexual individuals of past generations, gender non-conforming youth and adults today remain subject to diagnosis of psychosexual disorder and resulting social stigma and loss of civil liberty.

The Transvestic Fetishism diagnosis is broadly opposed among the trans-community and advocates for many of the same reasons that the psychiatric diagnosis of homosexuality was deemed inappropriate.

However, there is a second issue to the diagnosis of Gender Identity Disorder that differs from prior issues of homosexuality diagnosis. For the portion of the trans-community who is transsexual and painfully distressed by physical sex characteristics or birth-assigned gender role (a distress known as gender dysphoria), access to hormonal or surgical transition procedures is a matter of medical necessity. There is a need for some kind of diagnostic coding to facilitate access to this care, and the GID diagnosis is currently utilized by supportive care providers for this purpose.

It seems paradoxical that medical professionals who are affirming of their transitioning clients are forced to dispense a

3

diagnostic label that is derogatory toward them. In truth, supportive providers have to make do with a flawed diagnostic nomenclature whose criteria contradict transition. GID is currently defined to favor gender-reparative therapies: attempting to change one's inner gender identity or suppress one's outer gender expression. Although the APA denies that the DSM is intended to suggest treatment methods, this bias is evident in the diagnostic criteria, supporting text and placement in the manual. For psychiatric clinicians with intolerant views of gender diversity, this diagnosis provides a blunt instrument to enforce conformity to birth-assigned gender role. Consequently, the current GID diagnosis poses barriers to medical care related to corrective hormonal and surgical transition procedures: barriers that supportive medical and mental health professionals are compelled to overcome.

These dual issues of social stigma for all gender transcendent people, and medical necessity of transition procedures for those who need them, have divided trans-people and mental health providers alike on the GID diagnosis. This division has suppressed dialogue and forward progress in mental health policy for many years. Some advocates have called for immediate deletion of Gender Identity Disorder from the DSM-IV-TR. Others have reluctantly defended the diagnosis to maintain the present tenuous level of access to transition procedures for some.

My own view is that both issues of social stigma and medical necessity of transition are crucially important, and that we gender transcendent people have been wronged by the current GID diagnosis on both issues. I have long advocated reform of diagnostic nomenclature that addresses both issues and not one at the expense of the other.

Moreover, the removal of homosexuality from the DSM-III-R did not occur in a single step, but in incremental stages over a fourteen year span. Like a badly impacted molar, the diagnosis of homosexuality was excised painfully in pieces. "Sexual Orientation Disturbance" remained in the 7th printing of the DSM-II in 1974[6] and was renamed "Ego-dystonic Homosexuality" in the DSM-III in 1980.[7] This was finally removed from the DSM-III-R in 1987.[8] While these interim diagnostic categories were controversial, they served a purpose in facilitating forward progress. I expect that forward progress to reform or replace the GID diagnosis may require transitional diagnostic nomenclature as well.

The Fifth Edition of the *Diagnostic and Statistical Manual of Mental Disorders* (DSM-V) is presently under development by the APA for publication in 2012. It offers the first opportunity for revision of diagnostic categories and criteria in nearly two decades and possibly the last opportunity for two decades more. Although issues of access to transition medical care differ from those faced by Frank Kameny and gay dissidents in the 1970s, transgender issues of social stigma rooted in the *Diagnostic and Statistical Manual of Mental Disorders* are very similar. The issues of human dignity are very much the same.

In 2004, I had the opportunity to speak with Dr. Kameny at a convention of the National Gay and Lesbian Task Force, an organization he co-founded. I was inspired beyond words to hear his narrative of the events that led to changing policies and changing attitudes toward gay and lesbian people in American Psychiatry. He was quick to point out that times and tactics have changed since then. For those of us from the trans-community who have spoken at annual meetings of the APA, scholarship and refereed review have replaced fisticuffs as the price of admission, and for me that is a good thing. In the 1970s, however, the leadership of the American Psychiatric

5

Association was ready to listen and reconsider false stereotypes about sexual orientation. Dr. Kameny offered encouragement that attitudes in American psychiatry might change about gender diversity as well. He said, "You are on the verge of being heard."

This book contains a collection of essays from the struggle for transgender dignity and health care access. They are expanded from pieces posted to the GID Reform Advocates web site in 2008 and incorporate the generous feedback and discussion from advocates and critics.

The opinions expressed here are my own and do not necessarily represent those of other GID Reform Advocates.[9]

For students of psychology, sociology, anthropology and gender studies curricula, this book provides an overview of the literature and social context that led to the current diagnostic nomenclature. It offers a historical snapshot of the issues and challenges faced by the trans-community on the eve of publication of the DSM-V. For gender transcendent people, this book is a call for respect and celebration of the broad diversity that exists within our community. Yet, it is also a call for unity and solidarity in demanding change for psychiatric policies and stereotypes that dehumanize all trans-people. For mental health clinicians who work with transitioning clients, this book is intended to provide some insight, from a trans-perspective, into the barriers to social legitimacy and access to medical care that are posed by the present gender diagnoses in the DSM-IV-TR.

For policy makers involved with the DSM-V Task Force, this book is a plea to consider the consequences of the current Gender Identity Disorder and Transvestic Fetishism categories to the health, safety, civil justice and human dignity of gender transcendent people.

I hope that this book will encourage dialogue and understanding that lead to forward progress on reducing the terrible stigma of mental illness and sexual deviance that exists for all gender transcendent people and on reducing barriers to corrective medical and surgical care for those who need them.

Because our identities are not disordered.

[1] G. Speer, American Psychiatric Association, correspondence to Dr. Frank Kameny, July 17, 1963, http://www.kamenypapers.org/correspondence/letter-americanpsychologicalassoc-071763.jpg

[2] M. Meinke, "Zapping the Shrinks: May 3, 1971," The Rainbow History Project, http://www.rainbowhistory.org/apazap.htm

[3] R. Bayer, *Homosexuality and American Psychiatry, The Politics of Diagnosis*, Princeton University Press, 1981

[4] American Psychiatric Association, *Diagnostic and Statistical Manual of Mental Disorders*, Fourth Edition, Text Revision, Washington, D.C., 2000, pp. 574-575, 576-582.

[5] F. Kameny and B. Gittings, "Gay, Proud and Healthy," 1972, http://www.kamenypapers.org/correspondence/gayproudandhealthy.jpg

[6] American Psychiatric Association, *Diagnostic and Statistical Manual of Mental Disorders*, Second Edition, 7th Printing, Washington, D.C., 1974

[7] American Psychiatric Association, *Diagnostic and Statistical Manual of Mental Disorders*, Third Edition, Washington, D.C., 1980

[8] American Psychiatric Association, *Diagnostic and Statistical Manual of Mental Disorders*, Third Edition, Revised, Washington, D.C., 1987

[9] "Advocates for Reform of Transgender Psychiatric Classification," GID Reform Advocates, http://www.gidreform.org/advocate.html

Part I: Making Identities Disordered

And if the band you're in
starts playing different tunes,
I'll see you on the dark side of the moon

- *Pink Floyd, "Brain Damage" 1973*

The Focus of Pathology

Two weeks after the American Medical Association passed a historic 2008 resolution supporting health insurance coverage for gender-confirming endocrine and surgical care,[1] Dr. David Stevens of the Christian Medical & Dental Associations slurred these medically necessary procedures as "mutilation" by stereotyping transsexual women and men as mentally ill,

> "...mutilation of the body is wrong, and it's sad that these people have this psychological disorder -- but it should be treated from a psychological perspective,"[2]

Sadly, this derogatory stereotype is rooted in flaws of the classification of Gender Identity Disorder in the *Diagnostic and Statistical Manual of Mental Disorders* (DSM-IV-TR), published by the American Psychiatric Association (APA). Indeed, the focus of pathology in successive revisions of the DSM has shifted further from persistent distress with one's current or anticipated physical sexual characteristics or current ascribed gender role (gender dysphoria[3]) toward nonconformity with assigned birth sex[4]. Consequently, barriers to social legitimacy and access to transition related medical care remain insurmountable for many gender dysphoric individuals.

Gender identity disorders first appeared in the class of Psychosexual Disorders in the DSM-III[5] with more focus on gender dysphoria than today. The Transsexualism diagnosis was defined by a persistent sense of discomfort and inappropriateness about one's anatomic sex and desire to live as a member of the "opposite" (affirmed) sex. Gender Identity Disorder of Childhood was characterized by a strong and

11

persistent stated desire to be, or insistence that one is of, the other (affirmed) sex. For natal males only, diagnostic criteria included nonconformity to masculine gender stereotypes, disparaging feminine attributes.

In the DSM III-R[6] Gender Identity Disorders were moved out of Psychosexual Disorders to the class of Disorders Usually First Evident in Infancy, Childhood or Adolescence in recognition of gender identity origin in early life. Although this reclassification was a positive change, the diagnostic criteria for children were broadened to include gender role nonconformity for natal girls, such as "persistent marked aversion to normative feminine clothing". Worse yet, a new category was added, Gender Identity Disorder of Adolescence or Adulthood, Nontranssexual Type (GIDAANT), defined by discomfort about one's assigned birth sex and gender expression outside of the assigned role in fantasy or actuality. For the first time, non-transsexual gender-variant individuals, who were comfortable and well adjusted in cross-sex roles, were classified as mentally ill under a Gender Identity Disorder.

In the DSM-IV,[7] Gender Identity Disorders were once again classified as sexual disorders, now called Sexual and Gender Identity Disorders. This rekindled the stereotype of sexual deviance. A single expanded Gender Identity Disorder diagnosis combined the DSM-III categories of Transsexualism, Gender Identity Disorder of Childhood and GIDAANT. Unlike prior editions, the DSM-IV encouraged concurrent diagnoses of GID and Transvestic Fetishism (TF), making the stigma of fetishism a social issue for male-to-female transsexual women. Gender Dysphoria was obfuscated in criterion B by the phrase, "Or a belief that he or she was born the wrong sex." (See appendix A.) Thus, transitioned adults no longer gender dysphoric remained indelibly pathologized by their belief rather than their distress. Diagnostic criteria for children were again broadened to place a greater emphasis on nonconformity to social sex stereotypes. These implicated children with no evidence of gender dysphoria as mentally ill [8].

A well intended clinical significance criterion was added to GID, TF and most diagnoses in the DSM-IV, to require clinically significant distress or impairment to meet the accepted definition of mental disorder. Unfortunately, it failed to distinguish intrinsic distress of gender dysphoria from that caused by external societal prejudice and intolerance: what Dr. Evelyn Hooker termed "ego defensive" response[9]. Therefore, the clinical significance criterion failed to counter the stereotype that all gender variance is disordered. The criterion was brushed aside by Drs. Kenneth Zucker and Ray Blanchard (members of the Sexual and Gender Identity Disorders teams for the DSM-IV and DSM-V editions) as "muddled" and having "little import."[10] However this position contradicted the APA's definition of mental disorder:

> "a clinically significant behavioral or psychological syndrome or pattern that occurs in an individual and that is associated with present distress... or disability... or with a significantly increased risk of suffering, pain, disability, or an important loss of freedom... Whatever its original cause, it must currently be considered a manifestation of a behavioral, psychological, or biological dysfunction in the individual."[11]

The shift in focus from gender dysphoria to gender nonconformity in recent DSM editions has implicated a growing number of gender-variant people with mental disorder and sexual deviance who meet no standard of "dysfunction in the individual." It has exacerbated barriers to medical care and social intolerance. It has poorly served the purpose of diagnostic nomenclature given by the World Professional

13

Association for Transgender Health (WPATH) Standards of Care:

"The use of a formal diagnosis is often important in offering relief, providing health insurance coverage, and guiding research to provide more effective future treatments"[12]

In sharp contrast to the American Psychiatric Association policy, the American Medical Association reinterpreted GID in 2008 as "a serious medical condition" rather than mental or sexual disorder, characterized by distress rather than nonconformity to assigned birth role:

"a persistent discomfort with one's assigned sex and with one's primary and secondary sex characteristics, which causes intense emotional pain and suffering;"[1]

Moreover, the American Psychological Association Task Force on Gender Identity, Gender Variance and Intersex Conditions stated in 2006:

"Many transgender people do not experience their transgender feelings and traits to be distressing or disabling, which implies that being transgender does not constitute a mental disorder per se."[13]

In the DSM-V, there is opportunity for the American Psychiatric Association to realign with contemporary attitudes about gender diversity among its peer organizations, to refocus the GID diagnostic criteria on distress with physical sex characteristics or distress with assigned birth role or ascribed social role that are incongruent with inner gender identity. There is an opportunity for the APA to clarify in the supporting text and in public policy statement that, in the

14

absence of dysphoria, gender identity and expression that vary from assigned birth sex are not, in themselves, mental disorder.

[1] American Medical Association, "Resolution 122, Removing Financial Barriers to Care for Transgender Patients," http://www.ama-assn.org/ama1/pub/upload/mm/16/a08_hod_resolutions.pdf , June 2008.

[2] C. Butts, "Transgenderism -- purely psychological?" *OneNewsNow*, http://www.onenewsnow.com/Culture/Default.aspx?id=161948 , July 2, 2008.

[3] Working definition of Gender dysphoria by Dr. Randall Ehrbar and I following our panel presentations at the 2007 convention of the American Psychological Association. It is defined more ambiguously in glossary of the DSM-IV-TR as "A persistent aversion toward some of all of those physical characteristics or social roles that connote one's own biological sex." (p. 823)

[4] K. Winters, "Gender Dissonance: Diagnostic Reform of Gender Identity Disorder for Adults," *Sexual and Gender Diagnoses of the Diagnostic and Statistical Manual (DSM): A Reevaluation*, Eds. Dan Karasic, MD. and Jack Drescher, MD., Haworth Press, 2005; co-published in *Journal of Psychology & Human Sexuality*, Vol. 17 issue 3, pp. 71-89, 2005.

[5] American Psychiatric Association, *Diagnostic and Statistical Manual of Mental Disorders*, Third Edition, 1980, pp. 261, 263, 265.

[6] American Psychiatric Association, *Diagnostic and Statistical Manual of Mental Disorders*, Third Edition, Revised, 1987, pp. 71, 73, 76, 77, 424.

[7] American Psychiatric Association, *Diagnostic and Statistical Manual of Mental Disorders*, Fourth Edition, 1994, pp. 493, 536, 581.

[8] K. Winters, under pen-name K. Wilson, "The Disparate Classification of Gender and Sexual Orientation in American Psychiatry," *1998 Annual Meeting of the American Psychiatric Association*, Workshop IW57, Transgender Issues, Toronto, Ontario Canada, June 1998. This paper is a revised and expanded version of a previous article of the same title, published in *Psychiatry On-Line, The International Forum for Psychiatry*, Priory Lodge Education, Ltd., April, 1997, www.priory.co.uk/psych.htm. The original article is available on-line at www.priory.com/psych/disparat.htm.

[9] E. Hooker, E., "A Preliminary Analysis of Group Behavior of Homosexuals." *Journal of Psychology*. #41, p. 219, 1956

[10] K. Zucker and R. Blanchard, "Transvestic Fetishism: Psychopathology and Theory," in D. Laws and W. O'Donohue (Eds.), *Sexual Deviance: Theory and Application*, Guilford Press, New York, 1997, p. 258.

[11] American Psychiatric Association, *Diagnostic and Statistical Manual of Mental Disorders*, Fourth Edition, Text Revision, Washington, D.C., 2000, p. xxxi.

[12] World Professional Association for Transgender Health (formerly Harry Benjamin International Gender Dysphoria Association) "Standards of Care for Gender Identity Disorders," Sixth Version, http://wpath.org/Documents2/socv6.pdf , 2001

[13] American Psychological Association, "Answers to Your Questions About Transgender Individuals and Gender Identity," APA Task Force on Gender Identity, Gender Variance and Intersex Conditions, http://www.apa.org/topics/transgender.html, 2006.

A preliminary revision of this essay was posted at GID Reform Advocates: K. Winters, "Disordered Identities: The Focus of Pathology," July 7, 2008, www.gidreform.org/blog2008Jul07.html

The Disaffirmed Childhood

Jazz, a beautiful seven year old girl with long brown hair and poise beyond her years, explained gender diversity from her porch swing in a YouTube video this summer:

> "If someone asks me why I used to be a boy and now I'm a girl, I would say that I have a girl brain and a boy body. I think like a girl, but I just have a boy body and it's different than you."[1]

The American Psychiatric Association could have learned a lot from this young girl. Last year, Jazz and her family appeared with Barbara Walters in the television news magazine 20/20. They shared how painful her assigned birth-role had been for her until her family acknowledged her feminine identity at age five and created a safe space for Jazz to be herself. They shared how her distress was relieved with transition to a female social role and how she has thrived since.[2]

It is important to note that for preadolescent children, transition refers to a change in social gender role and not medical or surgical intervention. The earliest medical treatments, if needed, would come later at initial stages of puberty. According to endocrinologist Norman Spack, hormone blockers called GnRH analogues may be prescribed to delay onset of unwanted puberty and avoid resulting emotional trauma as well as "the physically and psychologically painful procedures required to reverse puberty's physical manifestations."[3]

In the context of children, transition is not assignment or coercion by parents or clinicians. Transition means simply creating an environment where gender-variant or transcendent[4] children may safely express their inner sense of gender identity without shame or fear. These roles may be stereotypically masculine, feminine or uniquely in between and may include self-expression in clothing and mannerisms and identification in name and pronouns. However, the APA labels all youth who transition their social gender roles as mentally disordered in the *Diagnostic and Statistical Manual of Mental Disorders, IV-TR* (DSM),[5] regardless of how happy and well they are in their new roles. Many of the barriers these youth face in school and society are exacerbated by these psychiatric labels. In the Byzantine language of the current Gender Identity Disorder in Children (GIDC) diagnosis, gender transcendent children should be closeted and neither seen nor heard.

In fact, gender role transition itself is misconstrued as symptomatic of psychosexual illness in the diagnostic criteria for GIDC. Of the four criteria for diagnosis,[6] the first is intended to address gender identity and is the most confusing and controversial:

Criterion A for Gender Identity Disorder in Children:

A strong and persistent cross-gender identification (not merely a desire for any perceived cultural advantages of being the other sex). In children, the disturbance is manifested by four (or more) of the following:

1. repeatedly stated desire to be, or insistence that he or she is, the other sex
2. in boys, preference for cross-dressing or simulating female attire; in girls, insistence on wearing only

stereotypical masculine clothing
3. strong and persistent preferences for cross-sex roles in make-believe play or persistent fantasies of being the other sex
4. intense desire to participate in the stereotypical games and pastimes of the other sex
5. strong preferences for playmates of the other sex

Of the five characteristics of criterion A, only the first has anything to do with gender identity and it is not required for diagnosis. The remaining four are based strictly on nonconformity to social birth sex stereotypes, and only four of the five characteristics are required. Thus, a child may be diagnosed with Gender Identity Disorder without evidence of gender identity that is incongruent with natal sex - without ever stating any desire to be the "other sex."

The last four characteristics pathologize, as mental illness and sexual disorder, behaviors and self-expression that would be considered ordinary for other children. In the supporting text of the GIDC diagnosis, these are described to include playing with Barbie dolls, homemaking and nurturing role play for birth-assigned males and aversion to cars, trucks, competitive sports and so-called "rough and tumble" play. For birth-assigned females, pathology is implied by playing Batman or Superman, competitive contact sports, and aversion to dolls or wearing dresses. Criterion A serves a punitive role in enforcing these dated, narrow and sexist gender stereotypes for children, upon penalty of diagnosis of mental disorder. The fifth characteristic, a "strong preference for playmates of the other sex" seems to equate mental health with sexual discrimination.[7]

In criterion A, birth-assigned males are inexplicably held to a much stricter standard of conformity than birth-assigned females in their choice of clothing and activities. A simple

21

preference for cross-dressing or "simulating" female attire meets the diagnostic criterion for the former but not for the latter, who must insist on wearing only male clothing to merit diagnosis. In modern Western culture, where children's clothing is often unisex, terms like "stereotypical" or "normative" seem archaic.[8]

In criterion A, "other sex," "cross-sex," and "cross-dressing," are defined with respect to assigned birth sex with no clarification regarding current affirmed gender role. This is evidenced in the criterion and supporting text, where children are always termed by birth sex pronouns, regardless of transition status. For example, an affirmed transitioned girl, such as Jazz, is maligned as a "boy" and "he" in the DSM. There is no exit from diagnosis for her or other transitioned youth who are happy and well adjusted in their affirmed gender roles; they will permanently meet criterion A as it is currently written.

Criterion B for Gender Identity Disorder in Children:

Persistent discomfort with his or her sex or sense of inappropriateness in the gender role of that sex. In children, the disturbance is manifested by any of the following:

- in boys, assertion that his penis or testes are disgusting or will disappear or assertion that it would be better not to have a penis, or aversion toward rough-and-tumble play and rejection of male stereotypical toys, games and activities;
- in girls, rejection of urinating in a sitting position, assertion that she has or will grow a penis, or assertion that she does not want to grow breasts or

menstruate, or marked aversion toward normative feminine clothing.

The second diagnostic criterion is intended to embody gender dysphoria, a term coined by Dr. Norman Fisk in 1973,[9] but profoundly misses its mark. From a Greek root for distress, gender dysphoria is defined here as a persistent distress with one's current or anticipated physical sexual characteristics or current ascribed gender role.[10] While a dated definition of gender dysphoria remains in the DSM-IV-TR glossary,[11] its meaning in the current criterion B is far less clear than in previous editions.

"Discomfort" and "inappropriateness" seem euphemistic in describing the intense and often debilitating distress that many children experience with their anatomy or assigned birth sex role. While the criterion describes elements of anatomic dysphoria,[12] it lacks clarity for distress with anticipated physical sex characteristics for preadolescent birth-assigned males, such as facial hair, voice change and upper body musculature. Most troubling, criterion B substitutes nonconformity to gender stereotypes for distress with assigned birth sex role. The phrases following the "or" in the sentences for "boys" and "girls," which include "rough-and-tumble play" and "normative feminine clothing," make criterion B redundant to criterion A. For example, children who are profoundly distressed by their birth sex assignment and corresponding names and pronouns are not clearly described in criterion B, while gender nonconforming youth with no clear evidence of anatomic dysphoria or distress with their assigned birth sex may be falsely implicated. Like the first criterion, there is no exit for children whose gender dysphoria has been relieved by social role transition. Transitioned youth permanently meet criterion B as it is currently written, even more so than before transition. Finally, criterion B fails to exclude discomfort from social intolerance as symptomatic of mental disorder.

Criterion C for Gender Identity Disorder in Children:

The disturbance is not concurrent with a physical intersex condition.

The DSM-IV Subcommittee on Gender Identity Disorders recommended at one point that individuals born with anatomical or chromosomal intersex conditions be included in the GID diagnoses for adults, adolescents and children,[13] as did previous editions of the DSM. However, the final decision was to exclude them from GID diagnosis and recommend diagnosis of Gender Identity Disorder Not Otherwise Specified.[14]

Criterion D for Gender Identity Disorder in Children:

The disturbance causes clinically significant distress or impairment in social, occupational, or other important areas of functioning.

The 1994 DSM-IV was significantly changed from prior editions with the addition of a clinical significance criterion to most diagnostic categories. Its purpose was to establish a definition of mental disorder and limit false positive diagnosis of those who do not meet that definition.[15] This policy change was controversial within mental health professions[16] and was particularly opposed by some members of the DSM-IV Subcommittee on Gender Identity Disorders. In an article on the Transvestic Fetishism diagnosis, Dr. Kenneth Zucker, chair of the present DSM-V Sexual and Gender Identity Disorders work group and Dr. Raymond Blanchard, chair of the DSM-V paraphilias subcommittee, dismissed the clinical significance criterion as "muddled" and having "little import."[17] This view conflicted with that of Dr. Darrel Regier, Vice Chair of the DSM-V Task Force:

> "We do not consider something a disorder unless there is a clearly defined description of this entity and there is clearly some significant dysfunction and distress associated with it,"[18]

The central flaw in criterion D for the GID in Children category is that it fails to distinguish distress and impairment caused by gender dysphoria from those resulting from societal prejudice or intolerance. Dr. Zucker notes, "the standard of impairment in children with GID has been their poor same-sex peer relations, with attendant social ostracism."[19] Thus, ego-syntonic or self-accepting gender-variant children who are victimized by prejudice at school meet criterion D only because of hate from others. Gender-variant children with healthy peer relations with children of the same gender identity also meet criterion D, because their friends are not of the same birth-assigned sex. This lack of clarity serves to promote gender-reparative psychotherapies that attempt to change gender identity and repress all gender expression not conforming to birth sex. Zucker continues,

> "I hope that the vagaries of the distress/impairment criterion do not dissuade clinicians from providing early therapeutic intervention"

Moreover, Drs. Zucker and Susan Bradley, who chaired the DSM-IV GID Subcommittee, invoked circular logic to cast all children diagnosed with GID as cognitively impaired. They claimed that diagnosed children were more likely to "misclassify their own gender, which ... surely must lead to confusion in their social interactions."[20] In other words, children who disagree with their birth-assigned roles were presumed impaired by fiat.

Are these children, in truth, misclassifying their gender or are they certain of it? Is it more likely that their psychiatric examiners are confused about the true gender of these children?

The current diagnostic criteria for Gender Identity Disorder of Childhood are broadly over-inclusive. They encourage false-positive diagnosis of gender nonconforming children having no significant distress of gender dysphoria, and they encourage diagnosis of mental illness on the basis of victimization from prejudice and intolerance. Authors of the GIDC diagnosis in the DSM-IV acknowledged that nearly 30% of children who did not meet the DSM-III criteria would meet the current criteria in the DSM-IV, based on changes to criterion A alone. This was based on the authors' data from the Toronto Centre for Addiction and Mental Health (CAMH), formerly the Clarke Institute of Psychiatry.[21]

While the American Psychiatric Association has emphasized that the DSM "does not provide treatment recommendations or guidelines,"[22] the GIDC diagnostic criteria are heavily biased in favor of gender-reparative therapies that attempt to change gender identity and expression differing from birth sex assignment. Children whose gender-variant expression is shamed into the closet by these treatments no longer meet criteria A,B or D, even if they continue to verbalize unhappiness and rejection of their birth sex assignment. (Criterion C, regarding concurrent intersex conditions, would not be relevant to gender expression or transition status in this example.)

26

Emerging supportive alternatives to gender-reparative interventions have very recently been termed "Gender Identity Actualization" by therapist Reid Vanderburgh.[23] Sadly, the diagnostic criteria for Gender Identity Disorder in Children contradict these affirming treatment approaches, including social role transition to relieve distress of gender dysphoria. Youth who are happy and well adjusted after transition to affirmed gender roles and who may experience intolerance at school continue to meet criteria A, B and D, even if they are not distressed by their anatomy. In fact, they are stereotyped as even more symptomatic of mental disorder, according to these criteria, than before transition.

According to the American Psychiatric Association, the purpose of the DSM includes facilitation of research and communication among clinicians and researchers.[24] However, the diagnostic criteria for Gender Identity Disorder in Children arguably bias research on the persistence of gender identity in youth. Follow-up studies of gender-variant children commonly use GIDC diagnosis to select the study sample and evaluate gender dysphoria or transsexualism later in adolescence or adulthood.[25] [26] Since children can meet the DSM-IV criteria for GIDC on the basis of gender role nonconformity with no stated anatomic dysphoria, it follows that rates of persistent dysphoria at follow-up could be vastly under-reported. The actual impact of this error on current published literature is unclear, as follow-up studies still partially rely on data from subjects selected under the DSM-III and III-R. Drs. Zucker, Bradley and others have acknowledged concerns that the DSM-IV criteria for GID of Childhood may "'scoop in' youngsters who show extreme cross-gender behavior but are not necessarily gender-dysphoric." For example, Zucker has suggested that,

"Because of the putative conflation of gender identity dysphoria and gender role behavior, particularly in the point A criterion, one could argue that reform of the criteria is called for." [27]

With the publication of the DSM-V, there is opportunity to address very serious shortcomings in the diagnosis of Gender Identity Disorder in Children. I hope that the Sexual and Gender Identity Disorders Work Group will clarify distress with physical sex characteristics (including those anticipated at puberty) and distress with birth sex assignment as the focus of new diagnostic criteria. I urge the Work Group to remove all references to gender expressions that differ from birth sex roles from the diagnostic criteria. Expressions that would be ordinary or even exemplary for all other youth do not constitute mental illness in gender-variant youth.

Back on Jazz's porch swing, the seven year old concluded,

"It's ok to be different, because it just matters who you are. It doesn't matter if you're different than anybody else. It just matters that you're having a good time and you like who you are."

We all might learn a lot from this young lady.

[1] Jazz, "7yr. old Jazz's thoughts on being a Transgender Child," http://www.youtube.com/watch?v=7S5usRgY720

[2] A. Goldberg and J. Adriano, "'I'm a Girl' -- Understanding Transgender Children," ABC News *20/20*, April 27, 2007, http://abcnews.go.com/2020/story?id=3088298&page=1

[3] N. Spack, "Transgenderism," *Lahey Clinic Medical Ethics Journal*, Fall 2005, http://www.lahey.org/newspubs/publications/ethics/journalfall2005/journal_fall2005_feature.asp

[4] I define transgender, gender-variant and gender transcendent in a broadly inclusive community sense: describing those whose inner sense of gender identity or outer gender expression transcend social gender stereotypes or differ from those associated with assigned birth sex. I prefer transgender as a term of social identity and the latter two as terms of human phenomena.

[5] American Psychiatric Association, *Diagnostic and Statistical Manual of Mental Disorders*, Fourth Edition, Text Revision, Washington, D.C., 2000.

[6] DSM-IV-TR, 2000, p. 581.

[7] K. Winters (under pen-name K. Wilson), "The Disparate Classification of Gender and Sexual Orientation in American Psychiatry," 1998 Annual Meeting of the American Psychiatric Association, Workshop IW57, Transgender Issues, Toronto, Ontario Canada, June 1998. This paper is a revised and expanded version of a previous article of the same title, published *in Psychiatry On-Line, The International Forum for Psychiatry*, Priory Lodge Education, Ltd., April, 1997, www.priory.com/psych/disparat.htm.

[8] Winters, 1998.

[9] N. Fisk, "Gender dysphoria syndrome. (The how, what, and why of a disease)," In D. Laub & P. Gandy (Eds.), *Proceedings of the second interdisciplinary symposium on gender dysphoria syndrome* , Stanford, 1973, pp. 7-14.

[10] Working definition of Gender dysphoria by Dr. Randall Ehrbar and I following our panel presentations at the 2007 convention of the American Psychological Association.

[11] DSM-IV-TR, 2000, App. C, p. 823. "A persistent aversion toward some of all of those physical characteristics or social roles that connote one's own biological sex."

[12] K. Zucker and S. Bradley, *Gender Identity Disorder and Psychosexual Problems in Children and Adolescents*, Guilford Press, 1995, pp. 21-22.

[13] S. Bradley, Ray Blanchard, et al., "Interim Report of the DSM-IV Subcommittee on Gender Identity Disorder," *Archives of Sexual Behavior*, Vol. 20, 4, p. 339.

[14] DSM-IV-TR, 2000, p. 582.

[15] American Psychiatric Association, *Diagnostic and Statistical Manual of Mental Disorders*, Fourth Edition, Washington, D.C., 1994, pp.xxi, 7.

[16] Spitzer R.L., Wakefield J.C. (1999). "DSM-IV diagnostic criterion for clinical significance: does it help solve the false positives problem?" Am. J. Psychiatry 156:1856-64 http://ajp.psychiatryonline.org/cgi/content/abstract/156/12/1856.

[17] K. Zucker and R. Blanchard, "Transvestic Fetishism Psychopathology and Theory," in D. Lays and W. O'Donohue, eds., *Sexual Deviance: Theory, Assessment, and Treatment*, Guilford, 1997, p. 258.

[18] B. Alexander, "What's 'normal' sex? Shrinks seek definition," MSNBC , May 22, 2008, http://www.msnbc.msn.com/id/24664654/.

[19] K. Zucker, "Commentary on Richardson's (1996) 'Setting Limits on Gender Health,'" *Harvard Rev Psychiatry*, vol 7, 1999, p. 41.

[20] Zucker & Bradley, 1995, p. 58.

[21] K. Zucker, R. Green, et al., "Gender Identity Disorder of Childhood: Diagnostic Issues," in T. Widiger, A. Frances, et al., *DSM-IV Sourcebook*, Am. Psychiatric Assoc., 1998, p. 511.

[22] American Psychiatric Association, "APA STATEMENT ON GID AND THE DSM-V, " http://www.psych.org/MainMenu/Research/DSMIV/DSMV/APAStatements/APAStatementonGIDandTheDSMV.aspx , May 23, 2008.

[23] R. Vanderburgh, "Appropriate Therapeutic Care for Families with Pre-Pubescent Transgender/Gender-Dissonant Children," to be published in *Child Adolesc Soc Work J*, 2008.

[24] DSM-IV, 1994, p. xxiii.

[25] K. Drummond, S. Bradley, M. Peterson-Badali, K. Zucker, "A follow-up study of girls with gender identity disorder," *Developmental Psychology*, Vol. 44, 1, Jan 2008, p. 34-45.

[26] Zucker & Bradley, 1995, p. 290-301.

[27] K. Zucker, "Gender Identity Disorder in Children and Adolescents," Annu. Rev. Clin. Psychol., Vol. 1, 2005. p. 17.9.

A preliminary revision of this essay was posted at GID Reform Advocates: K. Winters, "Disallowed Identities: The Disaffirmed Childhood" October 28, 2008, www.gidreform.org/blog2008Oct28.html

The Ambiguously Sexual Fetish

In January 2000, Peter Oiler, a married Louisiana truck driver for the Winn-Dixie grocery chain, was fired from his job after he came out of the closet to his boss,

> "I told him ... I'm not gay, I'm transgendered."
> "I told him I have a tendency to dress as a lady."[1]

A Winn-Dixie manager explained why Peter, an exemplary employee of more than 20 years, was terminated:

> "[Oiler] was doing something that was abnormal in most people's opinion about what was accepted for a person who is a man."[2]

Unfortunately, such derogatory public perceptions about cross-dressing and "abnormality" are promoted by the American Psychiatric Association in the current *Diagnostic and Statistical Manual of Mental Disorders IV-TR.*[3] The diagnostic category of Transvestic Fetishism casts gender nonconformity in clothing as mental disorder and sexual deviance. Its inclusion in the DSM-IV-TR begs the question, should a clothing disorder merit psychiatric classification? Is cross-dressing by born-males a psychosexual wardrobe malfunction or is it simply a facet of human diversity "ubiquitous throughout human history?"[4]

The term, transvestite, was coined by Magnus Hirschfeld in 1910 from Latin roots meaning to cross-dress. Transvestism in the DSM-III was renamed "Transvestic Fetishism" (TF) in the DSM-III-R[5]. The very title equates cross-dressing with sexual fetishism and social stereotypes of perversion. It sexualizes a diagnosis that does not clearly require a sexual context. In fact, Hirschfeld rejected fetishism as a diagnostic label for cross-dressing that represents self-expression, erotic or not, rather than erotic focus on clothing itself.[6]

Cross-dressing very often represents social expression and social identity. People who identify as cross-dressers make up a large portion of the emerging transgender movement. The oldest U.S. national support organization for heterosexual cross-dressers, the Foundation for Personality Expression, was founded by Virginia Prince in the 1960s and is now known as The Society for the Second Self or Tri-Ess.[7] Tri-Ess describes cross-dressers as "ordinary heterosexual men with an additional feminine dimension." Their vision emphasizes "Full personality expression, in a blending of both our masculine and feminine characteristics, in order to be all we can be."[8] However, the diagnostic criteria for Transvestic Fetishism ambiguously reduces this social expression of femininity by cross-dressing males to sexual deviance.

Criterion A for Transvestic Fetishism:

Over a period of at least 6 months, in a heterosexual male, recurrent, intense sexually arousing fantasies, sexual urges, or behaviors involving cross-dressing.[9]

Criterion A is grammatically ambiguous.[10] The phrase, "sexually arousing," could be interpreted to apply to only "fantasies" or to all three of "fantasies, sexual urges, or behaviors" with very different meaning. The first interpretation would implicate all recurrent cross-dressing behavior as sexual deviance. This interpretation is promoted in the *DSM-IV Casebook*,[11] which recommends a TF diagnosis for a male whose cross-dressing is not necessarily sexually motivated. The second would limit the diagnosis to sexually motivated cross-dressing, as did the DSM-

III-R,[12] and imply the ackward phrase, "sexually arousing sexual urges." Although labeled a "fetishism," it is not clearly stated whether or not cross-dressing must be sexual in nature to qualify for diagnosis.

Moreover, coincidence is conflated with causality in the phrase "behaviors involving cross-dressing," which requires no actual erotic motivation. This can imply that all cross-dressing by born-males is sexually motivated, whether it is or not. The resulting stereotype of sexual deviance is not limited to cross-dressers but disparages genderqueer individuals and transsexual women as well. Full-time transition to a female social role could be interpreted as "behaviors involving cross-dressing" and therefore presumed to be "fetishistic" under Criterion A.

In the past, transsexual and gender dysphoric individuals were specifically excluded from Tranvestic Fetishism diagnosis in the DSM-III-R[13] and this exclusion was removed in the DSM-IV. A major focus of the DSM-IV Subcommittee of Gender Identity Disorders was to allow concurrent diagnosis of GID and TF which was prohibited in previous editions.[14] A positive consequence of this change removed barriers to medical transition care for transsexual women who had been diagnosed as "transvestites." However, it also broadened the stigma of sexual paraphilia and deviance to include many transsexual women.

Diagnosis of Transvestic Fetishism is limited to heterosexual males in Criterion A. Curiously, women and gay men are free to wear whatever clothing they chose without a label of mental illness. This criterion serves to enforce a stricter standard of conformity for straight males than women or gay men. Its double-standard not only reflects the social privilege of heterosexual males in American culture, but enforces it.[15] One implication, derogatory to women, is that biological males who emulate women, with their lower social status, are presumed irrational and mentally disordered, while biological females who emulate males are not. A second implication stereotypically associates femininity and cross-dressing with male homosexuality and serves to punish straight males who transgress this stereotype.

Author Arlene Lev noted that the TF diagnosis is "more about sexist values and conflicts between individuals and society than they are about sexual disorders and human distress."[16] This violates the definition of mental disorder given in the DSM, which specifically exclude "conflicts between the individual and society" without clinically significant dysfunction.[17]

Criterion B for Transvestic Fetishism:

The fantasies, sexual urges, or behaviors cause clinically significant distress or impairment in social, occupational, or other important areas of functioning.

Distress and impairment became central to the definition of mental disorder in the DSM-IV,[18] where a generic clinical significance criterion was added to all Sexual and Gender Identity disorders, including Criterion B of Transvestic Fetishism. It was an attempt to prevent false-positive diagnosis of people who do not meet the definition of mental disorder.

Unfortunately, Criterion B does not specifically define distress or impairment for the TF diagnosis. It does not allow for the existence of healthy, well-adjusted male-identified heterosexual cross-dressers. Moreover, Criterion B makes no distinction between internal clinical distress and that caused by external prejudice and discrimination. Tolerant clinicians may infer that transgender identity or expression is not inherently impairing, but that societal intolerance and prejudice are to blame for the

36

distress and internalized shame that trans-people often suffer.[19] However, clinicians intolerant of gender diversity will infer the opposite: that cross-gender identity or expression by definition constitutes impairment, regardless of the individual's happiness or well-being.

Dr. Kenneth Zucker, chair of the present DSM-V Sexual and Gender Identity Disorders work group and Dr. Raymond Blanchard, chair of the DSM-V paraphilias subcommittee, were critical of including the clinical significance criterion for Transvestic Fetishism and dismissed it as "muddled" and having "little import." They reasoned that "individuals with TF who consult mental health professionals are presumably, in some respect, distressed or impaired by their condition."[20] This circular logic is even more concerning because, "... adolescents with TF rarely self-refer. The initiative is invariably on the part of an adult."[21] This implies that cross-dressing youth who are subjected to intolerance by parents or authorities are classed *a priori* as mentally disordered.

Ironically, the clinical significance critera for five other paraphilia diagnoses in the DSM-IV-TR, Exhibitionism Frotteurism, Pedophilia, Sexual Sadism and Voyeurism, were revised with more precise wording to limit inappropriate diagnosis.[22] The APA apparently had no such concern for false-positive diagnosis of gender nonconforming males who meet no definition of mental disorder.

In the supporting text of the Transvestic Fetishism diagnosis, behaviors that would be considered ordinary or exemplary for genetic women are presented as symptomatic of mental disorder on the basis of born genitalia and sexual orientation. These include collecting and wearing female clothes or undergarments, dressing entirely as females, wearing makeup, expressing feminine mannerisms and "body habitus," and appearing publicly in a feminine role.[23] It is not clear how these same behaviors can be pathological for people of one gender and not for another.

More disturbing, the supporting text lists "involvement in a transvestic subculture" among symptomatic "transvestic phenomena." Psychiatric diagnosis on the basis of social, cultural or political affiliation evokes the darkest memories of medical abuse in American and European history. For example, women suffragettes who demanded the right to vote in the early 1900s were diagnosed and institutionalized with a label of "hysteria."[24] Immigrants, Bolsheviks and labor organizers of the same era were labeled as socially deviant and mentally defective by psychiatric eugenicists.[25] In truth, transgender support organizations worldwide are a primary source of support, education and civil rights advocacy for gender-variant people, families, friends and allies. Their necessity is a consequence of social intolerance, not of mental deficiency.

The TF diagnosis is currently classified as a sexual paraphilia, defined in the DSM-IV-TR as

> "recurrent, intense sexually arousing fantasies, sexual urges, or behaviors generally involving 1) nonhuman objects, 2) the suffering or humiliation of oneself or one's partner, or 3) children or other nonconsenting persons"[26]

Sexual paraphilias in the DSM include such terribly stigmatizing disorders as Pedophilia, Exhibitionism, Fetishism, Frotteurism, Sexual Masochism, Sexual Sadism, and Voyeurism. This placement of the TF diagnosis serves to legitimize false stereotypes that unfairly associate cross-gender expression with criminal or harmful conduct. It serves to sexualize self-expression that is not necessarily sexually motivated.

Lacking a clear justification for the Transvestic Fetishism diagnosis, according to the definition of mental disorder in the current DSM, its authors resorted to the heteronormative presumption:

> "If the phylogenetic function of sexuality or eroticism is reproduction, and if its ontogenetic function is to enhance pair-bond formation and intimacy, then TF clearly is problematic at both levels of analysis."[27]

This is essentially the argument used to justify the classification of homosexuality in prior editions of the Diagnostic and Statistical Manual.[28-30] In proclaiming gender role nonconformity as mental illness, the authors of Transvestic Fetishism fail to mention the role of intolerance, prejudice and sex stereotyping as barriers to intimacy and pair-bonding in a species as diverse as ours. Indeed, the TF diagnostic category coerces adherence to sex stereotypes.

Speaking at the 2003 Annual Meeting of the American Psychiatric Association, Dr. Charles Moser noted, "Diagnoses should be removed if they cannot be shown to meet the definition of a mental disorder unambiguously and be substantiated by appropriate research." [31] Arlene Lev concurred for the case of Transvestic Fetishism:

> "transvestic fetishism is a normal human behavior transformed into a mental illness. ... it should not be listed in a manual of mental disorders."[32]

Perhaps Peter Oiler said it best,

"I'm tired of the closet. It's dark and musty and I want out! I want to settle some issues I have with myself. I want to tell everyone in my situation, 'you are not alone.' It doesn't make you a weirdo to put on a dress or pants."[33]

With publication of the DSM-V, it is time for the American Psychiatric Association to remove the anachronistic and sexist diagnosis of Transvestic Fetishism. Nonconformity to gender stereotypes is not mental illness.

[1] GenderPAC, "GenderPAC National News Interviews Peter Oiler," Feb 2001, http://www.gpac.org/archive/news/notitle.html?cmd=view&msgnum=0275

[2] K. Choe, American Civil Liberties Union, "Why We're Asking Courts and Legislatures for Transgender Equality, " *Where We Are 2003: The Annual Report of the ACLU Lesbian & Gay Rights Project*, Jan 2003, http://www.aclu.org/lgbt/transgender/12077pub20030101.html

[3] American Psychiatric Association, *Diagnostic and Statistical Manual of Mental Disorders*, Fourth Edition, Text Revision, Washington, D.C., 2000.

[4] V. Bullough and B. Bullough, *Cross Dressing, Sex and Gender*, Univ. of Pennsylvania Press, 1993, p. 18.

[5] American Psychiatric Associatio, *Diagnostic and Statistical Manual of Mental Disorders*, Third Edition, Revised, 1987, p. 288.

[6] M. Hirschfeld, The *Transvestites: An Investigation of the Erotic Drive to Cross Dress*[Die Tranvestiten], Leipzig: Sporh, 1910; trans. M. Lombardi-Nash, Promethius Books, 1991, p. 161.

[7] V. Prince, R. Ekins, and D. King, *Virginia Prince: Pioneer of Transgendering*, Haworth Press, 2005, pp. 7-8.

[8] The Society for the Second Self, Inc. , http://www.tri-ess.org/

[9] DSM-IV-TR, 2000, p. 575.

[10] K. Winters (published under pen-name Katherine Wilson) and B. Hammond, "Myth, Stereotype, and Cross-Gender Identity in the DSM-IV," Association for Women in Psychology 21st Annual Feminist Psychology Conference, Portland OR, 1996, http://www.gidreform.org/kwawp96.html.

[11] Spitzer, R., editor, *DSM-IV Casebook, A Learning Companion to the Diagnostic and Statistical Manual of Mental Disorders (fourth edition)*, American Psychiatric Press, 1994, pp. 257-259.

[12-13] DSM-III-R, 1987, p. 289.

[14] Bradley, S., et al. (1991). "Interim Report of the DSM-IV Subcommittee on Gender Identity Disorders," *Archives of Sexual Behavior*, Vol. 20, 1991, No. 4, p. 338.

[15] K. Wilson (former pen-name for Kelley Winters), "Gender as Illness: Issues of Psychiatric Classification," 6th Annual ICTLEP Transgender Law and Employment Policy Conference, Houston, Texas, July 1997. Reprinted in *Taking Sides - Clashing Views on Controversial Issues in Sex and Gender*, E. Paul, Ed., Dushkin McGraw-Hill, Guilford CN, 2000, pp. 31-38. http://www.gidreform.org/kwictl97.html

[16] A. Lev, *Transgender Emergence, Therapeutic Guidelines for Working with Gender-Variant People and Their Families*, Haworth Press, 2004, p. 171.

[17] DSM-IV-TR, 2000, p. xxxi.

[18] DSM-IV, 1994, p. xxi.

[19] G. Brown, "Cross-Dressing Men Often Lead Double Lives," *The Menninger Letter*, April, 1995, pp. 4-5.

[20] K. Zucker and R. Blanchard, "Transvestic Fetishism: Psychopathology and Theory," *Handbook of Sexual Deviance: Theory and Application*, Guilford Press, 1997, p. 258.

[21] K. Zucker and S. Bradley, "Gender Identity Disorder and Tranvestic Fetishism," eds. S. Netherton, et al., *Child and Adolescent Psychological Disorders, A Comprehensive Textbook*, Oxford Press, 1999, p. 386.

[22-23] DSM-IV-TR, 2000, p. 574.

[24] M. Mayor, "Fears and Fantasies of the anti Suffragists," *Connecticut Review* 7, No. 2, April 1974, pp. 64-74.

[25] I. Dowbiggin, *Keeping America Sane: Psychiatry and Eugenics in the United States and Canada, 1880-1940*. Sage House, 1997, pp. 133-177.

[26] DSM-IV-TR, 2000, p. 566.

[27] Zucker and Blanchard, 1997, p. 262.

[28] S. Rado, *Psychoanalysis of Behavior II*, Grune and Stratton, 1962.

[29] C. Socarides, *The Overt Homosexual*, Basic Books, 1962.

[30] R. Stoller, J. Marmor, I. Beiber, et al.,"A Symposium: Should Homosexuality be in the APA Nomenclature?" *American Journal of Psychiatry*, Vol. 130, 1973, pp. 1208-1215,

[31] C. Moser and P. Kleinplatz, "DSM-IV-TR and the paraphilias: An argument for removal." *Journal of Psychology and Human Sexuality* 17(3/4), also published in *Sexual and Gender Diagnoses of the Diagnostic and Statistical Manual (DSM)*, Eds. D. Karasic, and J. Drescher, Haworth Press, 2005, p. 106.

[32] Lev, 2004, p. 171.

[33] GenderPAC, 2001.

A preliminary revision of this essay was posted at GID Reform Advocates: K. Winters, "Disordered Identities, The Ambiguously Sexual Fetish" November 2, 2008, www.gidreform.org/blog2008Nov02.html

Maligning Language of Oppression

Of the disrespectful language faced by gender-variant people, none is more damaging or hurtful than that which disregards our gender identities, denies affirmed social roles of those who have transitioned, and reduces us to our assigned birth sex. I am speaking of affirmed transwomen called "he" and transmen called "she." I use the term Maligning Language to describe this specific kind of verbal violence.

In Colorado, Governor Bill Ritter signed a historic civil rights bill in May, 2008 extending public accommodation protection to transgender and gender nonconforming individuals. This legislation and the trans-community were quickly attacked by Dr. James Dobson and Focus on the Family in a hateful radio ad campaign that invoked the most painful false stereotypes of transwomen:

> "A man in a dress came into the girl's restroom at school today." [1]

Even worse, an innocent young affirmed Colorado girl was defamed and ridiculed this year by Denver NBC Affiliate KUSA-TV, because she dared to seek an education in a public elementary school, just like other girls.[2] The sensational headline,

> "Boy Wants to Return to School as a Girl," [3]

ignited an unprecedented firestorm of condemnation and backlash in the national press toward transitioned youth and their families.

Maligning language contradicts the social legitimacy of transitioned individuals. It denies their humanity and contributes to an environment of intolerance, discrimination and even physical violence. Tragically, such disrespectful conduct is encouraged with the authority of the American Psychiatric Association (APA) in the diagnosis of "Gender Identity Disorder" (GID) in the *Diagnostic and Statistical Manual of Mental Disorders IV-TR* (DSM).[4]

The very name, Gender Identity Disorder, implies "disordered" gender identity: that our identities are themselves disordered or deficient; that our gender identities are not legitimate, but represent perversion, delusion or immature development. In other words, the current GID diagnosis in the DSM-IV-TR implies that transwomen are nothing more than mentally ill men and maligns transmen as mentally ill women. This is repeated throughout the diagnostic criteria and supporting text for GID, where our affirmed identities and transitioned roles are termed "other sex" (with respect to assigned birth sex), and transsexual women are called "males," and "he." For example,

> "For some males …, the individual's sexual activity with a woman is accompanied by the fantasy of being lesbian lovers or that his partner is a man and he is a woman."[4]

Maligning language is repeated in scholarly literature by some of the most prominent authors of the current and pending gender diagnoses. Dr. Ray Blanchard of the Toronto Centre for Addiction and Mental Health (CAMH, previously known as the Clarke Institute of Psychiatry) introduced, "homosexual" and "non-homosexual" transsexualism, to sexology literature in 1989.[5] This language is so convoluted that it is hard to follow. Heterosexual transwomen attracted to men are labeled as "homosexual," reducing them to a stereotype of crazy gay "men." Lesbian or bisexual transwomen attracted to women or both are termed as "non-homosexual," again maligning all of them as "men." These labels leave no room for any non-pathologized sexuality for lesbian and bisexual transwomen.

Dr. Blanchard also labels this second group as "autogynephiliac," meaning a narcissistic love of one's self as a woman, a sexual paraphilia that he postulates to be the primary motivation for transition. This demeaning term is advanced in the supporting text for the GID diagnosis in the current DSM,[4] and there is broad concern within the trans-community that "autogynephilia" may be canonized as a new diagnostic category in the DSM-V [6].

Most shocking, Dr. Blanchard maligned all post-operative transsexual women with the following slur to a nationally distributed Canadian newspaper in 2004:

> "A man without a penis has certain disadvantages in this world, and this is in reality what you're creating." [7]

In May, Dr. Blanchard was appointed by the APA as Chairman of the Subcommittee for Paraphilias in the DSM-V Sexual and Gender Identity Disorders Work Group. He was also a member of the DSM-IV Subcommittee for Gender Identity Disorders.

I have found evidence that many mainstream medical and mental health professionals who work with the trans-community are moving away from maligning language. Reviewing presentation and poster abstracts from the 2007 Symposium of the World Professional Association for Transgender Health (WPATH), I counted over 90% of about 140 with language I considered gender neutral or gender affirming. The most positive examples used wording that was both respectful and clinically descriptive, such as

"transsexual women (post-operative male-to-female transsexuals on oestrogen replacement)."[8]

The most objectionable examples labeled research subjects by natal or assigned sex, regardless of gender identity, social gender role or hormonal or surgical status. For instance, straight transsexual women were maligned as

"Homosexual Transsexual South Korean Males"[9]

by primary author Dr. Kenneth Zucker, chairman of the DSM-V Sexual and Gender Identity Disorders work group and prior member of the DSM-IV Subcommittee for Gender Identity Disorders. While the latter practice represents the thinking behind the current GID diagnosis in the DSM-IV-TR, there are now many positive counterexamples in the literature to suggest alternative language for the DSM-V.

The influence of the DSM carries social consequences for all gender transcendent people, far beyond issues of mental health and medical care. Maligning terminology in the DSM enables and legitimizes defamatory social stereotypes like "a man in a dress," "a man without a penis," or "The Man Who Would be Queen" [10] in the press, the courts, the workplace and within families.

I implore all members of the DSM-V Task Force to consider the harmful consequences of maligning language in the current GID diagnosis and the future DSM-V.

[1] M. Zelinger, "Radio Ad Causes Anti-Discrimination Bill Controversy," News Channel 13, http://www.krdo.com/Global/story.asp?S=8362990 , May 21 2008.

[2] K. Winters, "Unprofessional Journalism at KUSA-TV Denver," http://ai.eecs.umich.edu/people/conway/TS/News/US/Kelly%20Winters %20letter%202-10-08.html , Feb 10 2008.

[3] N. Garcia, "Boy Wants to Return to School as a Girl,' KUSA-TV, http://www.9news.com/news/article.aspx?storyid=85989 , Feb 7 2008.

[4] American Psychiatric Association, *Diagnostic and Statistical Manual of Mental Disorders*, Fourth Edition, Text Revision, Washington, D.C., 2000, pp. 570, 577.

[5] R. Blanchard, "The Classification and Labeling of Nonhomosexual Gender Dysphorias," *Archives of Sexual Behavior*, Vol 18[4], Aug 1989, pp. 315-334.

[6] Z. Symanski, "DSM Section 302.85," *Bay Area Reporter*, V. 38, N. 25, http://ebar.com/news/article.php?sec=news&article=3021 , June 19 2008.

[7] J. Armstrong, "The Body Within: The Body Without," *The Globe & Mail*, p. F1, http://evalu8.org/staticpage?page=review&siteid=7950 , Toronto, June 12 2004.

[8] E. Elaut, et al., "Hypoactive sexual desire in transsexual women: prevalence and association with testosterone levels," WPATH 20th Biennial Symposium, Chicago IL, September 2007.

[9] K. Zucker, R. Blanchard, T. Kim, C. Pie, C. Lee, "Birth Order and Sibling Sex Ratio in Homosexual Transsexual South Korean Males: Effects of the Male-Preferring Stopping Rule," WPATH 20th Biennial Symposium, Chicago IL, September 2007.

[10] J. Bailey, *The Man Who Would Be Queen: The Science of Gender Bending and Transsexualism*, Joseph Henry Press, 2003.

A preliminary revision of this essay was posted at GID Reform Advocates: K. Winters, "Maligning Terminology: The Language of Oppression" June 24, 2008, www.gidreform.org/blog2008Jun24.html

Part II: Horns of a False Dilemma

Said the Cheshire Cat: 'We're all mad here.
I'm mad. You're mad.'

'How do you know I'm mad?' said Alice.

'You must be,' said the Cat,
'or you wouldn't have come here.

- *Lewis Carroll, 1865*

.

A False Dilemma

The trans-community has been divided by fear that we must choose between access to corrective hormonal and surgical procedures to support transition and the stigma of mental illness imposed by the current diagnosis of Gender Identity Disorder (GID).[1] This schism has allowed little dialogue and no progress on GID reform in nearly three decades. However, the GID diagnosis has failed gender-variant and especially transsexual people on both points. Transsexual individuals are poorly served by a diagnosis that stigmatizes them, before and after transition, as mentally deficient and sexually deviant and at the same time undermines the legitimacy of social transition and medical transition.

Gender Identity Disorder in the *Diagnostic and Statistical Manual of Mental Disorders IV-TR*[2] has imposed stigma of mental illness and sexual deviance upon people who meet no scientific definition of mental disorder[3]. It does not acknowledge the existence of many healthy, well-adjusted transsexual and gender-variant people or justify why all are labeled as mentally ill.

I have heard countless narratives of suffering inflicted by the stereotype of mental illness and "disordered" gender identity, and I have experienced it myself. We lose our families, our children, our homes, jobs, civil liberties, access to medical care and our physical safety. With each heartbreak, we're almost invariably told the same thing – that we're "nuts," that our identities and affirmed roles are madness and deviance. The following statement by Dr. Robert Spitzer at the 1973 annual meeting of the American Psychiatric Association remains as true today for transgender people as it was for gay and lesbian people then:

> "In the past, homosexuals have been denied civil rights in many areas of life on the ground that because they suffer from a "mental illness" the burden of proof is on them to demonstrate their competence, reliability, or mental stability."[4]

The current GID diagnosis places a similar burden of proof upon gender-variant individuals to prove their competence, with terrible consequences of social stigma and denied civil rights. It harms those it was intended to help. For example, the Vatican issued this directive in 2003 stating:

> "Transsexuals suffer from mental pathologies, are ineligible for admission to Roman Catholic religious orders and should be expelled if they have already entered the priesthood or religious life."[5]

Simultaneously, GID in the DSM-IV-TR undermines and even contradicts social transition and the medical necessity of hormonal and surgical treatments that relieve the distress of gender dysphoria (defined here as a persistent distress with one's current or anticipated physical sexual characteristics or current ascribed gender role[6]). For example, Paul McHugh, M.D., former psychiatrist-in-chief at Johns Hopkins Hospital, cited the GID diagnosis in 2004 as a key reason to eliminate gender-confirming surgeries:

> "I concluded that to provide a surgical alteration to the body of these unfortunate people was to collaborate with a mental disorder rather than to treat it."[7]

54

Dr. Paul Fedoroff of the Centre for Addiction and Mental Health (formerly the Clarke Institute of Psychiatry) cited the psychiatric diagnosis to urge elimination of gender-confirming surgeries in Ontario in 2000,

> "TS [transsexualism, in reference to the GID diagnosis] is also unique for being the only psychiatric disorder in which the defining symptom is facilitated, rather than ameliorated, by the 'treatment.' ... It is the only psychiatric disorder in which no attempt is made to alter the presenting core symptom."[8]

Paradoxically, the GID diagnosis has been defended as necessary for access to hormonal and surgical transition procedures. It is required by Standards of Care of the World Professional Association for Transgender Health[9], and GID is cited in legal actions to gain access to these procedures. Attorney Shannon Minter, head counsel for the National Center for Lesbian Rights was quoted in *The Advocate*,

> "'When we go to court to advocate for transsexual people to get medical treatment in a whole variety of circumstances, from kids in foster care to prisoners on Medicaid,' the GID diagnosis is used to show that treatment is medically necessary."[10]

Dr. Nick Gorton echoed longstanding fears that access to hormonal and surgical procedures would be lost if the GID were removed entirely,

> "Loss of the DSM diagnostic category for GID will endanger the access to care, psychological well being, and in some cases, the very life of countless disenfranchised

transgender people who are dependent on the medical and psychiatric justification for access to care."[11]

Gender dysphoric trans-people have therefore assumed that we must suffer degradation and stigma by the current GID diagnosis or forfeit lifesaving medical transition procedures. But has our community been impaled on the horns of a false dilemma?

Are hormonal and surgical procedures available to transitioning individuals because of the current diagnosis of "disordered" gender identity or in spite of it? Because the GID criteria and supporting text are tailored to contradict transition and pathologize birth-role nonconformity[3], affirming and tolerant professionals are burdened to re-construe GID in a more positive and supportive way for transitioning clients. For example, last month the American Medical Association (AMA) passed a historic resolution, "Removing Financial Barriers to Care for Transgender Patients." It reinterpreted GID to emphasize distress and de-emphasize difference:

> "... a persistent discomfort with one's assigned sex and with one's primary and secondary sex characteristics, which causes intense emotional pain and suffering."[12]

The AMA statement is perhaps a model for what the GID diagnosis should become in the DSM-V.

The current GID diagnosis and its doctrine of "disordered" gender identity have failed the trans-community on both issues of harmful psychosexual stigma *and* barriers to medical care access. The DSM-V Sexual and Gender Identity Disorders Work Group has an opportunity to correct both failures with new diagnostic nomenclature based on scientific standards of distress and impairment rather than intolerance of social role nonconformity and difference from assigned birth sex.

[1] This essay is expanded from K. Winters, "Harm Reduction for Gender Disorders in the DSM-V," Philadelphia Trans Health Conference, May 2008.

[2] American Psychiatric Association, *Diagnostic and Statistical Manual of Mental Disorders*, Fourth Edition, Text Revision, Washington, D.C., 2000.

[3] K. Winters, "Gender Dissonance: Diagnostic Reform of Gender Identity Disorder for Adults," *Sexual and Gender Diagnoses of the Diagnostic and Statistical Manual (DSM)*, Eds. D. Karasic, and J. Drescher, Haworth Press, 2005; co-published in *Journal of Psychology & Human Sexuality*, Vol. 17 issue 3, pp. 71-89, 2005.

[4] R. Spitzer, "A Proposal About Homosexuality and the APA Nomenclature: Homosexuality as an Irregular Form of Sexual Behavior and Sexual Orientation Disturbance as a Psychiatric Disorder," *American Journal of Psychiatry*, Vol. 130, No. 11, November 1973 p.1216

[5] N. Winfield, Associated Press, "Vatican Denounces Transsexuals," *Newsday*, Jan 2003.

[6] Working definition of Gender dysphoria by Dr. Randall Ehrbar and I following our panel presentations at the 2007 convention of the American Psychological Association. It is defined in glossary of the DSM-IV-TR as "A persistent aversion toward some of all of those physical characteristics or social roles that connote one's own biological sex." (p. 823)

[7] P. McHugh, "Surgical Sex," *First Things* 147:34-38, http://www.firstthings.com/ftissues/ft0411/articles/mchugh.htm , 2004.

[8] J. Fedoroff, "The Case Against Publicly Funded Transsexual Surgery," Psychiatry Rounds, Vol 4, Issue 2, April 2000.

[9] World Professional Association for Transgender Health (formerly HBIGDA), "Standards of Care for The Hormonal and Surgical Sex Reassignment of Gender Dysphoric Persons," http://wpath.org/Documents2/socv6.pdf , 2001

[10] S. Rochman, "What's Up, Doc?" *The Advocate*, http://www.advocate.com/issue_story_ektid50125.asp , Nov 2007.

[11] R.N. Gorton, "Transgender as Mental Illness: Nosology, Social Justice, and the. Tarnished Golden Mean," www.Nickgorton.org/misc/work/private_research/transgender_as_mental_illness.pdf , 2006.

[12] American Medical Association, "Resolution 122, Removing Financial Barriers to Care for Transgender Patients," http://www.ama-assn.org/ama1/pub/upload/mm/16/a08_hod_resolutions.pdf, June 2008.

A preliminary revision of this essay was posted at GID Reform Advocates: K. Winters, "Diagnosis vs. Treatment: Horns of a False Dilemma," July 01, 2008, www.gidreform.org/blog2008Jul01.html

Barriers to Medical Care

The psychiatric classification of gender variance as Gender Identity Disorder (GID) in the *Diagnostic and Statistical Manual of Mental Disorders* (DSM)[1] has long been cited as necessary to provide access to medical transition procedures for transsexual individuals who need them. According to Dr. Ira Pauly of the DSM-IV Subcommittee on Gender Identity Disorders,

> "Research in the field has been facilitated by having standardized criteria available for correctly diagnosing individuals with GID.... This has greatly increased our knowledge and understanding of GID, and has resulted in improved and more standardized treatment protocols."[2]

Standards of Care of the World Professional Association for Transgender Health continue to require a GID diagnosis for access to hormonal or surgical transition procedures[3]. Many fear that hormonal and surgical procedures might be withheld without some kind of diagnosis to validate their medical necessity and justify their risks. While the existence of *a* diagnostic coding has helped affirming, supportive care providers to make transition procedures available to some transitioning individuals, the specific diagnostic criteria and supporting text of the current Gender Identity Disorder category support the opposite approach – punitive gender-conversion or gender-reparative therapies intended to change or suppress gender identity or expression which differ from assigned birth sex roles[4].

61

However unintended, the consequences of the doctrine of "disordered" gender identity in the current DSM-IV-TR include barriers to medical care for transitioning individuals far beyond the scope of transition itself. The following examples of disparate health benefit coverage are common among large corporate employers[5] and would apply to transitioning intersex as well as transsexual employees. Similar barriers exist within government health benefits, small business health plans and private insurance policies.

Denied Coverage for Corrective Surgical Procedures

Transsexual individuals who suffer distress with their physical sex characteristics or ascribed social gender role (defined here as gender dysphoria[6]) are singled out by many employers and insurers for exclusion from coverage for corrective procedures that are commonly covered for cisgender or non-trans people.

Medically necessary surgical treatment for gender dysphoria does not necessarily require expanded or special coverage, but often employs the same or similar procedures already commonly covered for non-transsexual employees for a wide variety of congenital and endocrine conditions.[7]

Surgical Procedures Performed on Transsexual and Non-TS Individuals	Associated Conditions In Non-Transsexual Individuals
Vaginoplasty, Labia Construction	Congenital androgen insensitivity syndrome, Congenital adrenal hyperplasia, Vaginal agenesis, Vaginal atresia, Mayer-Rokitansky syndrome
Reduction mammoplasty, Chest Reconstruction	Gynecomastia
Metoidioplasty,	Congenital micropenis,

Scrotoplasty Urethral Extension	Congenital Buried Penis Syndrome, Epispadias, Hypospadias

These surgical procedures correct the same physiology and function for non-transsexual and transitioning individuals alike and are not broadly excluded in health benefits for those insured who are not transsexual. However, transitioning individuals are singled out by many insurers and employers for denial of coverage with a broad exclusion such as:

> "All expenses related to gender reassignment, including those related to complications arising from such services." [8]

This discrimination is based solely on gender identity, often in violation of corporate and state equal opportunity policies.

Denied Coverage for Endocrine Specialty Care

I have found much confusion around coverage for hormone replacement therapy (HRT) for gender dysphoric individuals or those who have completed physical transition. At my own employer, one woman was covered for HRT while employed, but then she was denied coverage under post-employment, or Cobra, benefit after she was terminated from employment.

Non-trans men and women who require HRT for treatment of androgen or estrogen deficiencies are covered under most benefit plans; while the same or similar treatment for transitioning individuals is explicitly excluded by many plans under the phrase, "All expenses related to gender reassignment."[8] Such policy can be used to prevent any transitioning or transitioned person from equitable access to hormone replacement therapy.

63

Denied Coverage for Conditions Prevalent among Females

Natal cisgender (non-trans) women are typically covered for a variety of conditions prevalent among women. However, affirmed women (male-to-female, or MTF) fear denial of coverage for conditions like breast cancer or osteoporosis by many insurers and employers, which exclude any conditions that might be construed as a "complication" of the transition process or hormone therapy. There is no assurance of equal coverage for these potentially fatal conditions.

Moreover, transitioning or affirmed men (FTM) may possess atypical physiology with the possibility of conditions prevalent among natal women, such as cervical or ovarian cancer. Transmen may be singled out for denial of coverage for these fatal conditions within many health plans for treatments "not appropriate based on the gender of the patient." [11] The award-winning documentary, *Southern Comfort* chronicles the tragic death of Mr. Robert Eads, a trans-man who was similarly refused treatment for ovarian cancer.[9]

Denied Coverage for Conditions Prevalent among Males

Conversely, natal men are typically covered for conditions unique or prevalent among men. However, affirmed men (FTM) may be denied treatment for conditions that are covered for other men if they are construed as "complications" of the transition process or hormone therapy.

Transitioning or transitioned women (MTF) may possess atypical physiology susceptible to conditions common to natal men, such as prostate cancer. While prostate cancer risk is much lower for transitioned women than natal men, cases have been reported[10], and regular examination and PSA screening are recommended.

Such care is currently denied under many benefit policies, which deems it "not appropriate based on the gender of the patient." [11]

Denied Mental Health Benefit Coverage

There is also a great deal of confusion about mental health care benefits for transitioning employees. Recognized medical standards of care for treatment of gender dysphoria and correction of physical sex characteristics are defined by the World Professional Association for Transgender Health (WPATH). While there is no scientific basis for casting gender diversity in itself as mental illness, anatomic dysphoria (persistent distress with one's physical sex characteristics[6]) is effectively treated with medical transition procedures.

However, the current standards require evaluation by a mental health professional with specialized knowledge of gender dysphoria and gender diversity issues prior to prescription of hormone replacement. For those who require surgical correction of sex characteristics, a period of 12 months of full-time "real-life experience" in their affirmed gender role is necessary for eligibility. An evaluation by a mental health professional is required for reduction mammoplasty and chest reconstruction for transmen, and evaluation by two mental health professionals is required for genital surgery eligibility for transmen and transwomen.[12]

However, benefit coverage for mental health evaluation and any psychotherapy specific to hormonal or surgical treatments may be denied under broad exclusions common to many insurers and employers, "All expenses related to gender reassignment."[8]

This exclusion could be used to deny any transitioning individual access to mental health assessments that are required by standards of care in the course of physical transition.

Maligning Stereotypes of Mental Illness

The only mental health benefits explicitly covered for gender dysphoric individuals under many health plans are those not "related to gender reassignment." Psychological treatments known as gender-conversion or gender-reparative therapies, which attempt to reverse innate gender identity or sexual orientation, fail to relieve distress of gender dysphoria and instead serve to shame gender-variant "patients" into the closet. Unfortunately, benefit coverage at many employers and insurers for these damaging psychotherapies, and simultaneous denial of hormonal and surgical medical care, combine to reinforce these defamatory stereotypes. The message implied by these benefits policies has contributed to a hostile work environment for many gender transcendent employees.

In recent years, a transsexual woman at my employer was mocked and ridiculed as mentally disordered by her supervisor, who told her,

> "I don't know why a 'man' would want to cross-dress. You know, the company will pay to fix this condition." [13]

She was terminated in the course of her transition.

The 2008 *Corporate Equality Index* [14] from the Human Rights Campaign surveyed 11,369 major U.S. businesses for policies and practices pertinent to GLBT employees, consumers and investors. Of these, less than one percent, 109, offered health benefit coverage for medically necessary surgical procedures to transitioning employees and their families.

The attitudes behind this epidemic transsexual health care discrimination are perhaps revealed by looking at those employers most publicized for their "equal opportunity" policies. The HRC awarded 195 employers with perfect 100% scores, denoting the very "best" workplaces for GLBT people. A disgraceful sixty percent of these, 117, specifically exclude transition surgical procedures. An important clue is found in nearly 80% of this group, 93, which cover "mental health counseling" for transitioning individuals while denying surgical benefits. Their intention to promote gender-conversion or gender-reparative psychotherapies in lieu of transition for those who suffer gender dysphoria seems clear.

In my view, this is evidence that prevalent transsexual health benefit discrimination is based on a false stereotype of "disordered" gender identity that equates gender difference with mental illness – a stereotype grounded in the DSM.

The current diagnosis of Gender Identity Disorder has contributed to derogatory stereotypes of mental illness and sexual deviance, creating barriers to medical care for transsexual and other gender-variant people before and after transition. The DSM-V Sexual and Gender Identity Disorders work group has an opportunity to refute these stereotypes with diagnostic criteria that do not conflict with social or medical transition and do not covertly promote punitive gender-reparative therapies.

[1] American Psychiatric Association, *Diagnostic and Statistical Manual of Mental Disorders, Fourth Edition*, Text Revision, Washington, D.C., 2000.

[2] I. Pauly, "Terminology and Classification of Gender Identity Disorders," *Interdisciplinary Approaches in Clinical Management*, New York: Haworth Press, 1992.

[3] World Professional Association for Transgender Health (formerly HBIGDA), "Standards of Care for The Hormonal and Surgical Sex Reassignment of Gender Dysphoric Persons," http://wpath.org/Documents2/socv6.pdf , 2001

[4] K. Winters, "Gender Dissonance: Diagnostic Reform of Gender Identity Disorder for Adults," *Sexual and Gender Diagnoses of the Diagnostic and Statistical Manual (DSM): A Reevaluation*, Ed. Dan Karasic, MD. and Jack Drescher, MD., Haworth Press, 2005; co-published in *Journal of Psychology & Human Sexuality*, Vol. 17 issue 3, pp. 71-89, 2005.

[5] Examples of health benefit inequity updated from K. Winters, "Issues of Transgender Health Benefit Inequity in the Corporate Equality Index," Seminar presented to the Human Rights Campaign, Washington, D.C., June 2008.

[6] Working definition of Gender dysphoria by Dr. Randall Ehrbar and I, following our panel presentations at the 2007 convention of the American Psychological Association. It is defined in glossary of the DSM-IV-TR as "A persistent aversion toward some of all of those physical characteristics or social roles that connote one's own biological sex." (p. 823)

[7] Thanks to Becky Allison, M.D., Gary Alter, M.D., and Marci Bowers, M.D., for input and information on these procedures and common health coverage practice. This table is far from exhaustive but illustrates examples of corrective surgical procedures, often denied to transsexual individuals, that are analogous to those covered for patients who are not transsexual. While not all health plans cover all of these procedures for cisgender (non-transitioning) individuals, broad exclusions to their coverage are not common.

[8] This language is used by my own employer, a Fortune 20 corporation, to deny coverage for all transition-related medical expenses in health plans administered by Aetna, UnitedHealthcare, and BlueCross BlueShield. It is

representative of common language I have heard in employee and private health plans.

[9] *Southern Comfort*, New Video Group, 2001. It may be viewed online at http://www.logoonline.com/shows/dyn/southern_comfort/videos.jhtml.

[10] R. Miksad, G. Bubley, et. al, "Prostate Cancer in a Transgender Woman 41 Years After Initiation of Feminization," Letter to the *Journal of the American Medical Assoc.*, v. 296 No. 19, Nov. 2006. http://jama.ama-assn.org/cgi/content/full/296/19/2316

[11] This language is currently used by UnitedHealthcare to exclude coverage of care for post-transition individuals at my employer that is unrelated to transition itself. It is representative of language I have heard in other employee and private health plans.

[12] World Professional Association for Transgender Health (formerly Harry Benjamin International Gender Dysphoria Association) "Standards of Care for Gender Identity Disorders," Sixth Version, http://wpath.org/Documents2/socv6.pdf , 2001.

[13] GID Reform Advocates, Advocates' Statements, http://www.gidreform.org/advocate.html.

[14] Human Rights Campaign, *Corporate Equality Index*, 2008. http://www.hrc.org/issues/workplace/cei.htm.

A preliminary revision of this essay was posted at GID Reform Advocates: K. Winters, "Diagnosis vs. Treatment: Barriers to Medical Care" August 8, 2008, www.gidreform.org/blog2008Aug08.html

.

Psychosexual Stigma

In the spring of 2003, I sat at a long table in the Grand Ballroom of the San Francisco Marriott with six men in suits and ties. The only woman, the only transperson, the only scholar who was not a psychiatrist or mental health professional, I was the emissary from the dark side of the moon.

We were presenting a symposium entitled, "Sexual and Gender Identity Disorders: Questions for the DSM-V"[1]. The moderators and organizers were Drs. Dan Karasic and Jack Drescher of the Association of Gay and Lesbian Psychiatrists, a division of the APA, who would later co-edit a book that followed[2]. On the left side of the table, Drs. Darryl Hill and Charles Moser joined me in advocating reform of the Gender Identity Disorder (GID) and paraphilia diagnoses in the next *Diagnostic and Statistical Manual of Mental Disorders*[3], published by the APA. At the far right end of the table, former APA President Dr. Paul Fink and Dr. Robert Spitzer, Chair of the DSM-III and DSM-IIIR Task Forces and editor of the *DSM-IV Casebook*[4], defended the status quo.

After formal presentations from the left and rebuttals from the right, Dr. Fink uttered a remark that stunned clinicians in the audience who were supportive of their transitioning clients. Speaking of the GID diagnosis, he said,

> "I think transsexualism is a diagnosis. ... And it certainly doesn't stigmatize anybody worse than the stigma they get every single day."[5]

71

Nearly five years later, I stood in a private school classroom in a conservative suburb where self-esteem was marked by enormous SUVs crowded between sprawling homes. The room was packed with angry parents and nervous staff. A group of us, consultants on gender diversity issues, had been asked to speak to their fears. A stranger in a strange land, a courageous young girl with a loving family had transitioned to her affirmed gender role in their midst.

One by one, voices around the room maligned this child and condemned her parents, threatening to remove their own children from the school if she was not expelled. As we tried to calm their panic, a hand shot in the air from one of the dominant males in the crowd, his eyes red with rage. He demanded the other parents reject this innocent girl, hissing through clenched teeth,

> "This is nothing more than mental illness, and the American Psychiatric Association says so."

This was far from the first time that the diagnoses of Gender Identity Disorder and Transvestic Fetishism by the APA had been cited to justify intolerance and discrimination. Virtually every aspect of transitioned life is impacted by these stereotypes of mental incompetence and sexual deviance. Gender transcendent people are denied medical care, child custody, housing, employment, and public accommodation as a consequence. Their very humanity in public discourse is dismissed as, "That's nuts."[6]

In 2007, the Maryland Montgomery County Public Schools introduced a health education curriculum including a lesson on "Respect for Differences in Human Sexuality" with an introduction to gender diversity. In a lawsuit against the school district, opponents to the curriculum rallied around the current gender disorders in the DSM:

> "the human sexuality lessons inaccurately portray 'transgender' as a 'sexual variation' when, transgenderism, gender dysphoria, and gender identity disorder actually constitute mental illness. American Psychiatric Association's Diagnostic and Statistical Manual of Mental Disorders (DSM-IV)."[7]

Fortunately, the circuit court decided in favor of the school district, but the same political extremists used the GID nomenclature to attack the Montgomery County gender identity nondiscrimination bill in November, 2007. A public notice from a group named Citizens for a Responsible Curriculum railed,

> "You can stop this! The vote on this bill is November 13th. Urge the Montgomery County Council to exclude entry into female restrooms, showers and dressing rooms by male transgenders and vice versa. The American Psychiatric Association recognizes Gender Identity Disorder as a mental illness."[6]

They ridiculed basic civil rights in public accommodation for gender-variant people, invoking sensational maligning headlines of transitioned women as deviant males. The Montgomery County board passed the bill, but legal and public attacks continued to rely on the authority of the American Psychiatric Association. For example, a Maryland political group dedicated an entire web page to denouncing transgender civil rights based on the DSM. It stated,

> "'Gender Identity Disorder' is classified as a mental disorder by the American Psychiatric Association. Legal

protection against discrimination based on mental illness is not provided for any other disorder, and there is no rational explanation why it should be offered for this one. Those who wish to assume a 'gender identity' contrary to their biological sex are in need of mental health treatment to overcome such disturbed thinking, not legislation to affirm it."[8]

The GID and TF diagnoses are used by national as well as local political and religious groups to promote intolerance of gender-variant people and even children. For example, in an article entitled "A Gender Identity Disorder Goes Mainstream" the influential Traditional Values Coalition (TVC) attacked the California Student and Violence Prevention Act of 2000[9] by invoking the mental illness stereotype:

> "In essence, this law gives sexually disturbed students the 'right' to self-identify their gender despite the biological reality of male and female. Under California state law, a boy who thinks he's really a girl, is now protected from alleged 'discrimination.' "[10]

They continued, "Gender confused individuals need long-term counseling, not approval for what is clearly a mental disturbance." The article cited the DSM to support the TVC's derogatory characterizations, "Transgenders are mentally disordered. The American Psychiatric Association (APA) still lists Transsexualism and Transvestism as paraphilias or mental disorders in the Diagnostic and Statistical Manual (DSM-IV-TR)"[10].

Contrary to Dr. Fink's denial of the problem, the role of psychiatric classification in perpetuating social stigma of mental incompetence and sexual deviance for gender-variant individuals has been long recognized by scholars and clinicians across academic disciplines. Anthropologist and author Anne Bolin noted in 1988, "The transsexual is labeled mentally ill and ipso facto in need of psychiatric care. ... The problems of stigma and the possible impact of the mental illness label are overlooked."[11]

More recently, clinical social worker Arlene Istar Lev, author of *Transgender Emergence*, concluded, "Reform of the GID diagnosis is necessary or the basic civil liberties for transgendered and transsexual people will remain elusive."[12] Drawing parallels between the current GID diagnosis and the past classification of homosexuality in the DSM, psychologist Madeline Wyndzen observed, "I find that the mental illness label imposed on transsexuality is just as disquieting as the label that used to be imposed on homosexuality."[13]

The American Psychiatric Association itself has acknowledged the potential harm of social stigma associated with a label of mental illness:

> "Scientific data cannot be interpreted in a vacuum. Sociological and other considerations must also be taken into account. ...we must consider instead how to balance the advantages of including the diagnosis in the DSM (e.g., increased detection of a treatable disorder with consequent reduction in morbidity and cost to the patient, his or her family, and to society at large) against the risks of making a false positive diagnosis (e.g., risk of stigmatization, cost and potential morbidity of unnecessary treatment, etc.)." [14]

Undermining the legitimacy of social and medical transition in the title, diagnostic criteria and supporting text of the current Gender Identity Disorder diagnosis, the American Psychiatric Association has undermined the human dignity and civil justice of gender-variant and especially transitioning people. The Sexual and Gender Identity Disorders work group of the DSM-V Task Force has an opportunity to reconsider consequences of social stigma that have been overlooked in past editions. It is time for diagnostic nomenclature that does not harm those it is intended to help.[15]

[1] K. Housman, "Controversy Continues to Grow Over DSM's GID Diagnosis," *Psychiatric News*, Vol. 38 No. 14, July 2003. http://pn.psychiatryonline.org/cgi/content/full/38/14/25 . I was listed under pen-name Katherine Wilson in this article. My presentation is summarized in K. Winters, "Gender Dissonance: Diagnostic Reform of Gender Identity Disorder for Adults," *Sexual and Gender Diagnoses of the Diagnostic and Statistical Manual (DSM): A Reevaluation*, Eds. D. Karasic, and J. Drescher, Haworth Press, 2005; co-published in *Journal of Psychology & Human Sexuality*, Vol. 17 issue 3, pp. 71-89, 2005. http://www.haworthpress.com/store/ArticleAbstract.asp?sid=DNFVJBXTS F848HQDMD0RDQAW67U17LP1&ID=67230

[2] D. Karasic and J. Drescher, Eds., *Sexual and Gender Diagnoses of the Diagnostic and Statistical Manual (DSM), A Reevaluation*, Haworth Press, 2005.

[3] American Psychiatric Association, *Diagnostic and Statistical Manual of Mental Disorders, Fourth Edition*, Text Revision, Washington, D.C., 2000.

[4] R. Spitzer, R., ed., *DSM-IV Casebook, A Learning Companion to the Diagnostic and Statistical Manual of Mental Disorders* (fourth edition). American Psychiatric Press, 1994.

[5] P. Fink, P., "Sexual and Gender Identity Disorders Discussion of Questions for DSM-V," *Journal of Psychology & Human Sexuality*, Vol. 17, Nos. 3-4, February2006, pp. 117-123, http://www.ingentaconnect.com/content/haworth/jphs/2006/00000017/F0 020003/art00008.

[6] Citizens for a Responsible Curriculum, "Public Notice," Damascus MD, November 2007, http://www.mcpscurriculum.com/pdf/transgender_alert.pdf

[7] Citizens for a Responsible Curriculum, et al. v. Montgomery County Public Schools, et al., Petitioners' Memorandum, Civil Action No. 284980, Circuit Court for Montgomery County, MD, October 2007, p. 10, http://www.mcpscurriculum.com/pdf/Appellate_Brief_PFOX2.pdf

[8] Maryland Citizens for a Responsible Government, "Referendum to Repeal Bill 23-07," Gaithersburg MD, http://www.notmyshower.net/gender_identity.shtml

[9] Gay-Straight Alliance Network, "AB 537 Fact Sheet, California Student and Violence Prevention Act"
http://www.gsanetwork.org/ab537/pdf/AB537.pdf

[10] Traditional Values Coalition, "A Gender Identity Disorder Goes Mainstream
Cross-dressers,Transvestites,And Transgenders Become Militants In The Homosexual Revolution," Anaheim CA, pp. 2-3,
http://www.traditionalvalues.org/pdf_files/TVCSpecialRptTransgenders1234 .PDF

[11] A. Bolin, *In Search of Eve*, Bergin & Garvey, South Hadley MA, 1988. p53.

[12] A. Lev, *Transgender Emergence, Therapeutic Guidelines for Working with Gender-Variant People and Their Families*, Haworth Press, 2004, p. 180.

[13] M. Wyndzen, M. H. "A Personal and Scientific look at a Mental Illness Model of Transgenderism." *American Psychological Association Division 44 Newsletter*, Spring 2004,
http://www.GenderPsychology.org/autogynephilia/apa_div_44.html

[14] American Psychiatric Association, "DSM-IV Frequently Asked Questions,"
http://www.psych.org/MainMenu/Research/DSMIV/FAQs/WhatistheDSM andwhatisitusedfor.aspx

[15] K. Wilson (former pen-name for Kelley Winters), "Gender as Illness: Issues of Psychiatric Classification," 6th Annual ICTLEP Transgender Law and Employment Policy Conference, Houston, Texas, July 1997. Reprinted in *Taking Sides - Clashing Views on Controversial Issues in Sex and Gender*, E. Paul, Ed., Dushkin McGraw-Hill, Guilford CN, 2000, pp. 31-38.
http://www.gidreform.org/kwictl97.html

A preliminary revision of this essay was posted at GID Reform Advocates: K. Winters, "Diagnosis vs. Treatment: Psychosexual Stigma" August 14, 2008, www.gidreform.org/blog2008Aug14.html

Part III: Blinded Me With Science

"It is not the butterfly's place to lecture the entomologist; it may feel pain whilst being pinned to a corkboard, but it had best keep that to itself."

Élise Hendrick, National Women's Studies Association Conference, 2008

Sampling Error

On May 28th, 2008, the American Psychiatric Association issued a "Statement on GID and the DSM-V" that emphasized,

> "The APA's goal is to develop a manual that is based on sound scientific data..."[1]

Has the APA, however, met this standard with the Gender Identity Disorder diagnosis in the current edition IV-TR of the *Diagnostic and Statistical Manual of Mental Disorders?*[2] Where are the "sound scientific data" to suggest, as do the title, diagnostic criteria and supporting text of the GID category, that gender-variant identities and expressions are intrinsically "disordered?"

The eminent physicist Bertrand Russell said of the scientific method:

> "A habit of basing convictions upon evidence, and of giving to them only that degree of certainty which the evidence warrants, would, if it became general, cure most of the ills from which this world is suffering."[3]

The cornerstone of empirical science is elimination of bias by sampling data that is representative of the population under study. Unfortunately, the APA's record for scientific vigor in the DSM is spotty. For decades, the classification of same-sex orientation as mental disorder was justified by research of subjects limited to clinical populations. Psychologist Evelyn Hooker noted in 1957 and earlier that gay and lesbian people

81

seeking psychiatric help or incarcerated in prisons and hospitals
did not constitute representative populations.

> "…few clinicians have ever had the opportunity to
> examine homosexual subjects who neither came for
> psychological help nor were found in mental hospitals,
> disciplinary barracks in the Armed Services, or in prison
> populations. It therefore seemed important, when I set
> out to investigate the adjustment of the homosexual, to
> obtain a sample of overt homosexuals who did not come
> from these sources."[4]

Astonishingly, another 16 years passed before psychiatric policy
makers began to take note. Psychiatrist Judd Marmor, urging
removal of homosexuality from the DSM in 1973, argued,

> "if our judgment about the mental health of heterosexuals
> were based only on those whom we see in our clinical
> practices we would have to conclude that all
> heterosexuals are also mentally ill."[5]

The authors of the GID diagnosis in the DSM-IV and current
revision IV-TR employed similarly unrepresentative data to
conclude that all gender-variant people, whose gender identity or
expression vary from their assigned birth sex roles, are mentally
disordered. For example, the GID authors relied upon their own
clinical populations from the "Sissy Boy" studies at UCLA[6] and
the Clarke Institute of Psychiatry (currently the Centre for
Addiction and Mental Health, CAMH, in Toronto) in developing
the diagnostic criteria for children:

> "Currently, the authors are analyzing data sets from
> Green's (1987) study and from the database of the Child
> and Adolescent Gender Identity Clinic at the Clarke

82

Institute of Psychiatry, Toronto, Canada, to examine the similarities and differences between children referred for gender identity concerns who do and do not verbalize the wish to be of the opposite sex." [7]

Moreover, clinical populations in mental health care, at least in the case of transvestic fetishism, were pre-judged *a priori* as impaired by Drs. Kenneth Zucker and Ray Blanchard of CAMH, members of the Sexual and Gender Identity Disorders Work Groups for the DSM-IV and DSM-V editions. They stated in 1997 that individuals, "...who consult mental health professionals are presumably, in some respect, distressed or impaired by their condition." [8] Their reasoning seems strangely reminiscent of Alice's experience in Wonderland:

"Said the Cheshire Cat: 'We're all mad here. I'm mad. You're mad.'

'How do you know I'm mad?' said Alice.

'You must be,' said the Cat, 'or you wouldn't have come here.'" [9]

What of non-clinical populations of gender-variant people? There is little evidence that follow-up studies, suggesting overwhelmingly positive outcomes for transsexual individuals whose gender dysphoria had been relieved by transition and corrective surgeries, were considered by the GID authors in the DSM-IV. [10] A unique controlled 1990 study of the benefit of genital surgery for (MTF) transsexual women by Mate-Kole, et al. [11], and a comprehensive 1992 review of 80 case studies spanning 30 years by Pfäfflin and Junge [12] are absent from the *DSM-IV Sourcebook* citations. Pfäfflin and Junge concluded that, "... we found most of the desired changes in the areas of partnership and sexual experience, mental stability and socio-economic functioning level." This data would have been helpful in refuting stereotypes of inherent psychological pathology that were embodied in the GID diagnostic criteria and supporting text.

To gain "sound scientific data," it is necessary to understand the demographics of the population under study in order to access its members. To this end, the DSM-IV-TR cites the prevalence of GID as, "... roughly 1 per 30,000 adult males and 1 per 100,000 adult females seek sex-reassignment surgery." These estimates are based on studies by Wålinder[13] and Hoenig[14] in the 1960s and 70s of patients who sought help in gender clinics in Sweden and the U.K. Last year, Professors Femke Olyslager and Lynn Conway presented an analysis to the World Professional Association for Transgender Health (WPATH) that revealed startling flaws in these figures[15]. For example, prevalence in the Hoenig study is understated by more than a factor of six, based on the study's own data, if the relevant general populations of birth-assigned males and females are corrected for appropriate age. Moreover, these studies rely on non-representative institutional samples of transsexual people, excluding all those who receive care from supportive private practitioners.

Aggregating a number of earlier studies, and accounting for general population demographics and conflation of prevalence with incidence in the early years of available surgical treatments, Olyslager and Conway reported that the prevalence of corrective surgical transition procedures was much higher than previously acknowledged in psychiatric literature. Their re-analysis of data from prior studies suggests a lower bound of 1:2900 to 1:5800 of the total population that has had or will have corrective surgery in support of transition, and they reported an even higher rate based on data from surgeons. Dr. Mary Ann Horton independently reported a similar surgical prevalence of 1:3100 per lifetime among US citizens.[16] As only a subset of transsexual individuals require or obtain surgical treatment, Olyslager and Conway went on to estimate the lower bound on prevalence of transsexualism at 1:500.[15] Moreover, transsexual individuals represent a subset of those meeting the current diagnosis of Gender Identity Disorder in the DSM-IV-TR, which relies heavily on gender role nonconformity rather than specific distress or incongruence with assigned birth sex.

These recent studies raise a crucial question, how can the American Psychiatric Association claim that the current GID diagnosis is based on "sound scientific data," representative of the gender-variant population, when they are unaware of the existence of as much as 99% of that population? Conway noted,

> "Such a truly egregious error presents a direct challenge to the psychiatric profession's credibility in the entire area of transsexualism."[17]

Where is this hidden silent majority of gender-variant people who are not to be found in clinical populations? Conway has compiled a collection of photos and stories for over 200 transitioned transsexual man and women living full lives, ordinary and extraordinary:

> "They are successes in living 'life in the large.' We see it in the happy faces, and sense it in between the lines of their stories. These are the successes of women who have survived and corrected their earlier transsexualism, and gone on to find joy and comfort and peace in their lives."[18]

We transsexual people are only the tip of the iceberg of gender-variant adults and youth currently implicated as mentally ill. In more than two decades that I have been active in the trans-community, I have been honored to meet hundreds of remarkable individuals who defy anachronistic stereotypes of mental impairment: people who have transitioned into very ordinary conventional male and female roles and into unique roles that defy convention, people who live in "stealth," quietly assimilated into society, and those who are out and proud as advocates and role models. I have heard their narratives, stories of grace and courage in the face of adversity that would likely overwhelm most other people. I have met countless real people in the real world with little resemblance to the doctrine of "disordered" gender identity perpetuated in the current DSM-IV-TR.

I hope that policy makers in the American Psychiatric Association will meet them too.

What Dr. Evelyn Hooker noted of gay men a half-century ago is perhaps even more true for gender-variant individuals today:

> "But what is difficult to accept (for most clinicians) is that some homosexuals may be very ordinary individuals, indistinguishable, except in sexual pattern, from ordinary individuals who are heterosexual. Or - and I do not know whether this would be more or less difficult to accept - that some may be quite superior individuals, not only devoid of pathology (unless one insists that homosexuality itself is a sign of pathology) but also functioning at a superior level."[4]

The current diagnosis of Gender Identity Disorder in the DSM-IV-TR allows no possibility for the existence of countless well-adjusted transsexual and gender-variant people already in society. The Sexual and Gender Identity Disorders work group has an opportunity to replace stereotypes with science in the DSM-V, to base diagnostic nomenclature on sound data that is representative of real gender-variant people from non-clinical populations.

[1] American Psychiatric Association, "APA Statement on GID and the DSM-V," http://www.psych.org/MainMenu/Research/DSMIV/DSMV/APAStatements/APAStatementonGIDandTheDSMV.aspx , May 23, 2008.

[2] American Psychiatric Association, *Diagnostic and Statistical Manual of Mental Disorders*, Fourth Edition, Text Revision, Washington, D.C., 2000, p. 579.

[3] Bertrand Russell, http://www.skepticreport.com/medicalquackery/camufo.htm

[4] E. Hooker, E., "The Adjustment of the Male Overt Homosexual," *Journal of Projective Techniques*, #21, p.18, 1957.

[5] R. Stoller, J. Marmor, I. Beiber, et al.,"A Symposium: Should Homosexuality be in the APA Nomenclature?" *American Journal of Psychiatry*, Vol. 130, pp. 1208-1209, 1973.

[6] R. Green, The *"Sissy Boy Syndrome" and the Development of Homosexuality*, Yale University Press, New Haven CT, 1987.

[7] T. Widiger, et al., eds., *DSM-IV Sourcebook*, Vol. 3, American Psychiatric Association, 1997, p. 320.

[8] K. Zucker and R. Blanchard, "Transvestic Fetishism: Psychopathology and Theory," in D. Laws and W. O'Donohue (Eds.), *Sexual Deviance: Theory and Application*, Guilford Press, New York, 1997, p. 258.

[9] Charles Dodgson (Lewis Caroll), *Alice's Adventures in Wonderland*, 1865.

[10] Note: One post-operative follow-up study cited in the *DSM-IV Sourcebook* by Blanchard, et al., was cited to support a remark in the text of the DSM-IV and DSM-IV-TR that transsexual women attracted to other women and transitioning in adulthood are "less likely to be satisfied after sex-reassignment surgery."(p. 580) This statement has posed barriers to surgical transition care for transsexual women, maligned as "males" in the supporting text, on the basis of their sexual orientation. R. Blanchard, B. Steiner, L. Clemmensen, R. Dickey, "Prediction of Regrets in Postoperative Transsexuals," *Can. J. Psychiatry*, 34, pp.43-45, 1989.

[11] C. Mate-Kole, M. Freschi , and A. Robin, "A controlled study of psychological and social change after surgical gender reassignment in selected male transsexuals." *Brit J Psychiat* 157: pp. 261-264, 1990.

[12] F. Pfäfflin and A. Junge , *Sex Reassignment: Thirty Years of International Follow-Up Studies after SRS -- A Comprehensive Review, 1961-1991,* 1992, English translation 1998, http://209.143.139.183/ijtbooks/pfaefflin/1000.asp.

[13] J. Wålinder, Incidence and Sex Ratio of Transsexualism in Sweden , *British Journal of Psychiatry*, Vol. 119, pp. 195-196, 1971.

[14] J. Hoenig and J.C. Kenna, "The prevalence of transsexualism in England and Wales,"
British Journal of Psychiatry, Vol. 124, pp. 181-190, 1974.

[15] F. Olyslager and L.Conway, "On the Calculation of the Prevalence of Transsexualism," WPATH 20th International Symposium, Chicago, Illinois, 2007.
http://ai.eecs.umich.edu/people/conway/TS/Prevalence/Reports/Prevalence%20of%20Transsexualism.pdf , Submitted for publication in the *International Journal of Transgenderism* (IJT).

[16] M. Horton, "The Cost of Transgender Health Benefits," Transgender at Work, http://www.tgender.net/taw/thbcost.html

[17] L. Conway, "The Numbers Don't Add; Transsexual Prevalence," http://www.gidreform.org/gid30285.html .

[18] L. Conway, "Transsexual Women's Successes: Links and Photos," http://ai.eecs.umich.edu/people/conway/TSsuccesses/TSsuccesses.html ; "Successful TransMen: Links and Photos," http://ai.eecs.umich.edu/people/conway/TSsuccesses/TransMen.html

A preliminary revision of this essay was posted at GID Reform Advocates: K. Winters, "Blinded Me With Science: Sampling Error" July 21, 2008, www.gidreform.org/blog2008Jul21.html

Devolution of the DSM

At the 2003 Annual Meeting of the American Psychiatric Association, Dr. Robert Spitzer, Chair of the DSM-III and DSM-III-R Task Forces, defended the categories of Gender Identity Disorder (GID) and paraphilias such as Transvestic Fetishism (TF) in the *Diagnostic and Statistical Manual of Mental Disorders* (DSM).[1] He declared that gender identities which vary from assigned birth sex are inherently disordered:

> "Children normally develop a sense of gender identity. It is not taught—it just happens. I would argue that by itself, the failure to develop a gender identity that is congruent with biological gender is a dysfunction."[2]

Spitzer based this premise not on empirical data but upon a theory of evolutionary essentialism, "the view that some 'things' (such as human beings) have properties or qualities that are invariable and represent the true essence of the 'thing.'" In this context, Spitzer defined a medical disorder as "some biological function that is expected—that is part of being a human being – that is not working." He disparaged gender-variant identities and expressions as pathological, because they do not serve what is "expected," because they are incongruent to a perceived biological function of the born body. Who, however, gets to decide what is "expected?" From whose perch of social privilege is American psychiatry to pass judgment upon the evolutionary worthiness of a class of people who have survived since human antiquity?

Dr. Spitzer's reasoning is very reminiscent of essentialist theories that upheld the classification of same-sex orientation as mental illness in previous editions of the DSM.[3] In the early 1960s, psychoanalyst Dr. Sandor Rado stated that "every individual is either male or female," based on reproductive anatomy, and that the only healthy sexual adaptation is male-female pair bonding[4]. Dr. Charles Socarides, co-founder of the anti-gay National Association for Research and Therapy of Homosexuality (NARTH), asserted that, "heterosexual object choice is determined by two and a half billion years of human evolution."[5] Psychoanalyst Dr. Irving Bieber echoed these views of biological heteronormativity. Arguing to retain homosexuality as a diagnosis in the DSM, he stated, "humans born with normal gonads and genitals are biologically programmed for heterosexual development."[6]

Ironically, Dr. Spitzer was himself instrumental in removing the diagnosis of homosexuality from the DSM between 1973 and 1987 and was strongly opposed by Socarides and his NARTH cohorts. Spitzer refuted essentialist arguments for homosexual pathology, noting that the purpose of the DSM is to list disorders, not human functioning that is judged "less than optimal." He explained,

> " if failure to function optimally in some important area of life, as judged by either society or the profession, is sufficient to indicate the presence of a psychiatric disorder, then we will have to add to our nomenclature the following conditions: celibacy (failure to function optimally sexually), revolutionary behavior (irrational defiance of social norms), religious fanaticism (dogmatic and rigid adherence to religious doctrine), racism (irrational hatred of certain groups), vegetarianism (unnatural avoidance of carnivorous behavior), and male

92

chauvinism (irrational belief in the inferiority of women)."[6]

Stanford evolutionary biologist Dr. Joan Roughgarden challenged assumptions of adaptive unfitness for gender diversity in her 2004 book, *Evolution's Rainbow: Diversity, Gender, and Sexuality in Nature and People.*[7] She concluded,

> "Diversity allows a species to survive and prosper in continually changing conditions,"

emphasizing that the occurrence of sexual and gender diversity across species and its prevalence among human beings across many cultures are inconsistent with stereotypes of pathology.

Roughgarden cited many examples of animal and plant species with more than two distinct genders and others with abilities to change sex from female to male and vice versa. A tropical ginger plant can change sex mid-day, making pollen in the morning and receiving pollen in the afternoon. A coral reef fish, the bluehead wrasse, has three genders, including large and small types of males. The larger type begins life as female and is aggressive toward the smaller males born male. A male clown fish can turn into a female, and hamlets, producing both sperm and eggs, switch roles several times as they mate. Gobies can crisscross sexes several times in their lives to relieve shortages of males or females. Forty-two species of hummingbirds exhibit "transgender expression," with females having masculine coloration and characteristics and vice-versa.

Regarding sexual orientation, Roughgarden cited ninety-four bird species known to mate in same-sex pairs. Geese can mate for life in male-male pairs, with some couples documented together over fifteen years. (A span that most American heterosexual couples might envy.) Male and female homosexual behavior has been found in over 100 mammalian species, including wild and domestic sheep, hyenas, kangaroos, squirrels, seals, sea lions, dolphins and whales. Among primates, bonobos (along with chimpanzees) are our closest genetic relatives. Male and female same-sex encounters are very common for bonobos, and they even use a set of hand signals to communicate the kind of sex they wish.

Among humans, Dr. Roughgarden proposed that transsexualism occurs too frequently to be explained by random mutation pruned by natural selection alone and therefore does not imply significant adaptive disadvantage. In 2007, Professors Femke Olyslager and Lynn Conway estimated the lower bound on prevalence of transsexualism at around 1:500, based on mathematical correction of prior studies and survey of surgical data[8], nearly 100 times greater than figures cited in the DSM.[1] Roughgarden noted that these estimates are consistent with those from the U.K and the Hijra in India of around 1:1000. She compared the prevalence of transsexualism to a 99.9 percentile score on a college entrance exam or an IQ of 130, stating that such relatively common traits "can only be consistent with a tiny and undetectable loss of fitness."[7]

Is social Darwinism in American psychiatry rooted in science or social bias? At the 2003 APA meeting, Dr. Spitzer echoed evolutionary psychologists who seemed to project rigid contemporary sex stereotypes (dominant, hunting males vs. passive, nurturing, gathering females) upon ancestral cultures.[9-10] He speculated:

> "In all cultures, young boys want to play with boys, Young girls want to play with girls... If you are interested in evolutionary psychology, you ask yourself could that

94

have some survival value? The answer is yes. Thousands of years ago when men were more likely to be in hunting and women were more likely to be in the nurturing role, if you were a young boy you would do better if you spent your time with other boys with whom, when you were older, you would go to the hunt."[2]

He went on, "...in all cultures, gender is recognized as a dichotomy."

To the contrary, anthropological research has revealed a long list of non-European cultures with more than two recognized sex and gender roles. Traditions of social gender role transition independent of birth sex include the Tahitian and Hawaiian Mahu, The Madagascar Sekrata, Hindu Tantric and Hijra Sects, Islamic Xanith, Khawal, and Sufi Traditions and others.[11-14] Gender diversity and fluidity was prominent in Greco-Roman mythology and culture and paradoxically coexisted with scriptural proscription in Western religious traditions.[15] Native American scholars now use the term Two Spirit to describe sex and gender traditions, common among First Nations, that are beyond dichotomy.[16]

In Colorado, Two-Spirit women (male-to-female), such as the Navajo Nadle, the Lakota Winkte and the Cheyenne He man eh,[17] held respected roles in healing and spiritual leadership. Gender transcendence was not only a normal variation of human life but sacred, a sign of a person especially close to the spirits. As a young boy, the great Chief Crazy Horse of the Lakota Sioux was blessed by a Winkte shaman in a secret naming ceremony. Possessing a secret Winkte name marked social status and conferred spiritual protection, good health and long life. Later, he married at least one Winkte wife, in addition to his wives born female.[14]

95

Like the blue wrasse fish, these proud Native American nations thrived for millennia, apparently unaware of any "adaptive disadvantage." That was, until European intolerance appeared on the plains in the form of the Seventh Cavalry and compulsory missionary and reservation schools, which drove these ancient traditions into the closet.[14] Among human societies, the anomaly is not the existence of gender diversity but the repression of it, isolated to mostly Western cultures, including our own. It seems astonishing that such a large, relevant body of social science has been ignored by previous authors of the *Diagnostic and Statistical Manual of Mental Disorders.*

In our modern global economy, as among the native nations of the Colorado plains, humans live and compete in communities. Adaptation and survival mean success of the tribe, perhaps more than individual breeding. Economist Richard Florida stated that in today's world, "Human creativity is the ultimate economic resource." In his book, *The Rise of the Creative Class,*[18] he tracked the growth of the "creative class," those doing creative work for a living, from less than 10 percent in 1900 to nearly a third in the year 2000 – a class generating as much wage and salary income as the manufacturing and service sectors combined. Surprising to many, he found strong correlations between the most diverse US communities and those with the highest creative class share. Five of the top ten metropolitan regions ranked for diversity, Seattle, Boston, Minneapolis, San Francisco, Austin, and Denver, also ranked in the top ten of creative class share. Four of these, San Francisco, Austin, Seattle and Boston, were in the top five regions for gay and lesbian population share, a component of the diversity ranking. And three of these, San Francisco, Boston and Seattle respectively, were the top three regions for high-technology industry. Dr. Florida concluded that lowering barriers to inclusion fosters creative ecosystems –

"Habitats open to new people and ideas, where people network easily and offbeat ideas are not stifled but are turned into new projects, companies and growth. Regions and nations that have such ecosystems are likely to do the best job of tapping the diverse creative talents of the most people, and thus gain competitive advantage."

Although Florida's analysis utilized gay and lesbian census data, where gender-variant populations are not counted, gender transcendent people are a vibrant and increasingly visible component of lesbian, gay, bisexual, transgender (GLBT) and straight communities – especially in urban centers. For example, of the top ten large metropolitan regions for creative class share in Florida's survey, seven prohibit employment discrimination based on gender identity - according to the Human Rights Campaign. These include Washington, D.C., Boston, Austin, San Francisco, Minneapolis, Denver, and Seattle. Nine of the top ten high-technology communities, all but Phoenix, have trans-inclusive civil rights ordinances.[18-19] Lowering barriers to gender diversity in these communities is associated with creative human capital and economic potential.

While correlation does not imply causality, there is growing evidence that gender diversity is far from a "dysfunction" in human communities. Diversity of gender identity and expression can contribute adaptive advantages in unique breadth of perspective and creative viewpoint to the cultural and economic success of communities, ancestral and modern.

Derogatory stereotypes that equate gender diversity with evolutionary unfitness and psychiatric pathology, like those of same-sex orientation that preceded them, are contradicted by the pervasive reality of gender diversity throughout nature and human culture. As Dr. Joan Roughgarden observed:

> "When scientific theory says something's wrong with so many people, perhaps the theory is wrong, not the people."[7]

I hope that the Sexual and Gender Identity Disorders work group of the DSM-V Task Force will reexamine the evidence that difference in itself is not disease.[16]

1 American Psychiatric Association, *Diagnostic and Statistical Manual of Mental Disorders, Fourth Edition*, Text Revision, Washington, D.C., 2000, p. 579

2 R. Spitzer, "Sexual and Gender Identity Disorders: Discussion of Questions for DSM-V," *Journal of Psychology & Human Sexuality*, Vol. 17, Nos. 3-4, February2006, pp. 111-116, http://www.ingentaconnect.com/content/haworth/jphs/2006/00000017/F0020003/art00008.

3 K. Winters (published under pen name Katherine Wilson), "The Disparate Classification of Gender and Sexual Orientation in American Psychiatry," 1998 annual meeting of the American Psychiatric Association, Workshop IW57, Transgender Issues, Toronto Canada, June 1998. http://www.gidreform.org/kwapa98.html

4 S. Rado, *Psychoanalysis of Behavior II*. New York: Grune and Stratton, 1962.

5 C. Socarides, *The Overt Homosexual*. New York: Basic Books, 1962.

6 R. Stoller, J. Marmor, I. Beiber, et al.,"A Symposium: Should Homosexuality be in the APA Nomenclature?" *American Journal of Psychiatry*, Vol. 130, pp. 1208-1215, 1973.

7 J. Roughgarden, *Evolution's Rainbow: Diversity, Gender, and Sexuality in Nature and People*, Univ. of CA Press, 2004, pp. 1, 21, 32-35, 102, 136-149, 282, 286-287,

8 F. Olyslager and L.Conway, "On the Calculation of the Prevalence of Transsexualism," WPATH 20th International Symposium, Chicago, Illinois, 2007. http://ai.eecs.umich.edu/people/conway/TS/Prevalence/Reports/Prevalence%20of%20Transsexualism.pdf , Submitted for publication in the *International Journal of Transgenderism* (IJT).

9 G. Alexander, "An Evolutionary Perspective of Sex-Typed Toy Preferences: Pink, Blue, and the Brain," *Archives of Sexual Behavior*, Vol. 32, 2003, 1991, pp. 7-17.

10 J. Benenson, "Sex Differences in Children's Investment in Peers," *Human Nature*, vol 9 no 4, 1998, pp. 369-390.

[11] C. Ford and F. Beach, F., *Patterns of Sexual Behavior.* New York, Harper and Brothers, 1951.

[12] A. Bolin, *In Search of Eve*, Bergin & Garvey, 1988.

[13] V. Bullough and B. Bollough, *Cross Dressing, Sex, and Gender*, University of Pennsylvania Press, 1983.

[14] W. Williams, *The Spirit and the Flesh: Sexual Diversity in American Indian Culture.* Boston, Beacon Press, 1986, pp. 37, 112. 177-196.

[15] A. Lev, Transgender Emergence: Therapeutic Guidelines for Working with Gender-Variant People and Their Families, Haworth Clinical Practice Press, 2004, pp. 62-67

[16] S. Jacobs, W. Thomas, S. Lang, *Two-Spirit People*, Univ of Illinois Press, 1997.

[17] K. Winters (published under pen-name Katherine Wilson) and B. Hammond, "Myth, Stereotype, and Cross-Gender Identity in the DSM-IV," Association for Women in Psychology 21st Annual Feminist Psychology Conference, Portland OR, 1996, http://www.gidreform.org/kwawp96.html.

[18] R. Florida, *The Rise of the Creative Class: And How It's Transforming Work, Leisure, Community and Everyday Life*, Basic Books, 2003, pp. xiii, xiv, xx, xxi, 244, 251.

[19] Human Rights Campaign, "Cities and Counties with Non-Discrimination Ordinances that Include Gender Identity" April 2008, http://www.hrc.org/issues/workplace/equal_opportunity/9602.htm.

A preliminary revision of this essay was posted at GID Reform Advocates: K. Winters, "Blinded Me with Science: Devolution of the DSM" August 20, 2008, www.gidreform.org/blog2008Aug20.html

The Burden of Proof

In the movie, *Ghostbusters*, Professor Peter Venkman, played by Bill Murray, deflected questions with a quip,

"Back off, man. I'm a scientist."[1]

In the reality of human gender diversity, the current diagnostic categories of Gender Identity Disorder (GID) and Transvestic Fetishism in the *Diagnostic and Statistical Manual of Mental Disorders IV-TR* (DSM) convey a presumption that internal gender identity or social gender expression that vary from assigned birth sex roles are intrinsically pathological and sexually deviant. Their authors and supporters have defended this axiom by disparaging criticism as an *attack* on science and academic expression. Thus, the premise of 'disordered' gender identity has ascended to the level of dogma in American psychiatry and psychology, imposing a near-impossible burden of proof upon contrary evidence, dissenting opinion and especially upon transitioned individuals to demonstrate their mental competence and their legitimacy in affirmed gender roles.

In an interview with MSNBC this year, Dr. Kenneth Zucker, chairman of the current DSM-V Sexual and Gender Identity Disorders Work Group and a chief author of the current GID diagnosis, stated that there "has to be an empirical basis to modify anything in the DSM."[2] However, has Dr. Zucker inverted the appropriate burden of proof here? Should his Work Group be equally committed to examine the validity of the current GID and TF diagnostic categories and the data used to justify them? What is the basis, where is the science to

101

substantiate the premise of 'disordered' gender identity that underlies these diagnoses?

Lilienfeld, Lynn and Lorh, editors of *Science and Pseudoscience in Clinical Psychology*, noted that,

> "the burden of proof in science rests invariably on the individuals making a claim, not on the critic."[3]

At the core of the GID diagnosis is the presumption that social or medical transition contrary to birth sex is always a negative outcome and acquiescence to birth sex role is a positive one. This is reflected in the diagnostic criteria, which tar even the happiest, most well adjusted post-operative transsexual men and women as permanently disordered, and absolve closeted or concealed gender dysphoria (distress with current physical sex characteristics or ascribed gender role) from diagnosis of mental illness[4]. This doctrine of 'disordered' gender identity is underscored throughout the supporting text, where persistent gender identity differing from birth sex is termed a "chronic course" of disorder and the need for gender congruence is disparaged as "preoccupation"[5].

In the *Treatment Companion to the DSM-IV-TR Casebook*, also published by the APA, gender-conversion or gender-reparative therapies, which attempt to change gender identity or expression that differ from birth sex, are recommended to clinicians for birth-role nonconforming and gender-dysphoric children, while supporting and affirming treatment approaches are excluded. In a chapter authored by Dr. Zucker, clinicians are advised to suspect parents in the "genesis and/or perpetuation of GID." Parents are told to "set limits" on gender role expression or even fantasy play nonconforming to birth sex, shaming their children into the closet. Successful outcome is only described in terms of "fading of ... cross-gender identification" and of being "helped so that the desire to change sex does not persist into adolescence and adulthood." Persistent (or un-closeted) gender identity or expression that differs from birth sex is cast as failure, with alarming predictions of social withdrawal and rejection by "both boys and girls."[6]

Zucker repeated these dire warnings to parents of gender-variant children in an interview on National Public Radio last May:

> "He explained that unless Carol and her husband helped the child to change his behavior, as Bradley grew older, he likely would be rejected by both peer groups. Boys would find his feminine interests unappealing. Girls would want more boyish boys. Bradley would be an outcast." [7]

Was this prediction based on science or just substitution of opinion as fact? In the same National Public Radio interview, Dr. Zucker's patient, "Bradley," was contrasted with a young girl, Jona, whose transition from male birth-role to female affirmed-role was supported by her parents and therapist, Dr. Diane Ehrensaft. Far from outcast or withdrawn, Jona's father described her as thriving:

> "She's so comfortable with her own being when she's simply left to be who she is without any of these restrictions being put on her. It's just remarkable to see."

Jona's case is far from unique. A growing number of parents and their affirming care providers are rejecting derogatory diagnosis and punitive conversion psychotherapies and are working with schools and communities to create safe spaces for their gender-variant children and adolescents to simply be themselves.

103

TransYouth Family Allies (TYFA), an education and support organization for gender-variant youth and families[8], has provided assistance to 125 families nationwide to date[9]. These children offer dramatic counter-examples to the DSM-IV-TR and its Treatment Companion text. For example, Boulder, Colorado pediatrician Dr. Jeff Richker describes a very positive outcome for an affirmed girl (MTF), who began her social role transition at age eight:

> "Lucia is 90 percent happier than Luc ever was … I think the transition has gone a long way to alleviating so much of the unhappiness in her life."[10]

Yet, the very existence of well adjusted, transitioned children is denied in the *DSM-IV-TR Treatment Companion* and subsequent literature, which denigrate real-life experience in affirmed gender roles as "fantasy solution". In their 1995 book, Drs. Zucker and Susan Bradley, previous Chair of the DSM-IV Subcommittee on Gender Identity Disorders, condemn affirming support of gender-variant children as therapeutic "nihilism," invoking a double-negative statement to justify gender-reparative psychotherapies: "we have found no compelling reason not to offer treatment to a child with gender identity disorder." Moreover, Zucker and Bradley insult the intelligence of all parents who reject or question gender-reparative therapies for their gender-nonconforming children: "Some parents, especially the well-functioning and intellectually sophisticated ones, are able to carry out these recommendations relatively easily and without ambivalence."[11]

Although Dr. Zucker concedes "that contrasex hormonal and surgical sex change may well be the best methods of treatment" for gender dysphoric adolescents, he casts this in a negative context of "much poorer" prognosis and failure of gender-conversion in earlier childhood. A derogatory view of nonconformity to assigned/birth sex roles is repeated in recent literature, coauthored by Zucker and Bradley, where "typical" and "normative" gender behavior are defined as synonymous. The authors incorrectly term persistence of masculine identity in birth-assigned girls as "persistence of gender dysphoria,"[12] obscuring the proven roles of social transition and medical treatment (the latter for adolescents and adults) in relieving distress with ascribed gender role and anatomical sex.

For adolescents suffering gender dysphoria, there is growing clinical evidence that social transition and postponement of adverse puberty (development of birth sex characteristics incongruent with inner identity) enable positive outcomes. In a 2007 presentation to the World Association for Transgender Health (WPATH), Dr. Annelou De Vries reports significant reduction of behavior and socialization problems for transitioned adolescents given puberty-blocking treatment, based on the Child Behavior Checklist (CBCL) and Youth Self-Report (YSL) assessment[13]. He notes "stable, improved psychological functioning" for these youth in contrast to the typecast of "much poorer" prognosis.

For adults, the myth of 'disordered' gender identity is also contradicted by co-morbidity studies that find a notable absence of psychopathology among transsexual individuals. In a large-scale 1997 study of 435 gender dysphoric subjects (318 MTF women and 117 FTM men), Cole, et al. concludes:

"This study should help to clear up certain misperceptions about gender dysphoria per se. Specifically, individuals presenting with gender dysphoria often do not have problems indicative of coexisting psychiatric illness such as schizophrenia or major depression. Instead, these findings suggest that gender dysphoria is usually an isolated diagnosis." [14]

While analogous findings about the mental health of gay men by Dr. Evelyn Hooker[15] were instrumental to the reform of the homosexuality diagnosis in the DSM-II and III, these analogous studies of gender-variant people have been largely disregarded by DSM policy makers. Studies of postoperative transsexual individuals from non-clinical populations also suggested positive outcomes for social role transition and corrective medical procedures to relieve distress of gender dysphoria in adults.[16-17] These data were corroborated by numerous positive post-transition narratives in print[18-21] and online,[22] evidence that seems to have been selectively overlooked in DSM policy.

In fact, clinicians and scholars with dissenting opinion and criticism of the GID and TF diagnoses have been met with hostility and personal insult themselves[23]. In her 1996 book *Gender Shock: Exploding the Myths of Male and Female* author Phyllis Burke described how the GID diagnosis was used to facilitate reparative therapy and hospitalization of gender non-conforming youth suspected of being "prehomosexual." She quoted Dr. Kenneth Zucker that parents bring children to gender clinics mostly "because they don't want their kid to be gay"[24]. In an interview for *Brain, Child* magazine, Zucker responded by attacking Ms. Burke *ad hominem*:

> "He dismisses her book as 'simplistic' and 'not particularly illuminating,' the work of a journalist whose views shouldn't be put into the same camp as those of scientists like Richard Green or himself."[25]

Such personal attacks are not limited to journalists. In a 1999 letter to the *Journal of Sex and Marital Therapy*, Dr. Zucker fired scathing insults at Richard Isay, M.D., who had raised similar concerns about the GID diagnosis for children in *Psychiatric News*.[26] Zucker stated, "one must raise the thorny and difficult question of Isay's professional credentials to comment on the validity of the diagnosis of gender identity disorder." Zucker called Dr. Isay's opinion "uninformed, both clinically and empirically" and his work "a cheap imitation of his predecessors."[27]

Negative stereotypes about transition outcomes are also refuted by the magnitude of post-transition and post-operative populations that integrate into society so completely that they remain undetectable to the psychiatric research establishment. Olyslager and Conway[28] presented evidence of mathematical flaws in earlier studies, suggesting that vastly more people have transitioned with corrective surgeries than figures cited in the DSM-IV-TR. Although their conclusions were independently corroborated in a health benefit cost analysis by Dr. Mary Ann Horton,[29] mental health policy makers in both American Psychiatric and Psychological Associations have ignored these challenges to longstanding belief about the prevalence of transsexualism. For example, a 2008 report from the American Psychological Association Task Force on Gender Identity and Gender Variance rejected Olyslager and Conway's work in a footnote, without bothering to examine their calculations or even list a citation to their paper. Just as disappointing, the American Psychological Association invoked guilt-by-association to discredit Olyslager and Conway, by claiming that their analysis was endorsed by "transgender activists."[30]

Suppressing dissent by labeling critics of derogatory psychiatric policies as transgender or transsexual "activists" is an unfortunate trend in recent mental health literature. For example, Dr. J. Michael Bailey, psychologist and author of, *The Man Who Would be*

Queen: The Science of Gender-Bending and Transsexualism,[31] and coauthor Kiira Triea panned critics of his controversial book and its underlying theory of "autogynephilia." Both the book and the theory, that all male-to-female transition is motivated by either homosexuality or narcissistic sexual paraphilia,[32] have evoked outrage among gender transcendent people.[33-34] In an article entitled, "What Many Transgender Activists Don't Want You to Know and Why You Should Know It Anyway," the authors maligned Bailey's critics *ad hominem* with labels of "nonhomosexual MTF transsexuals" and "autogynephiles in denial." Bailey and Triea exceeded the bounds of professionalism so far as to publicly speculate about the sexual orientations and private medical histories of people they had never met, including Becky Allison, M.D., Christine Burns, M.B.E., Professor Lynn Conway, Andrea James, Deirdre McCloskey, Ph.D., Nancy Nangeroni, and Joan Roughgarden, Ph.D. Their scorn also extended to clinicians who disagree with these derogatory depictions of transsexual women, describing supportive care providers as "colluding with autogynephiles in denial."[35]

Dr. Alice Dreger, a colleague of Bailey's at Northwestern University, voiced similar derogatory presumptions about the private sex lives and transitions of dissenting "transgender activists" in the *Archives of Sexual Behavior* (ASB). She stated, "women such as they might be labeled autogynephilic— individuals with paraphilias whose cross-sex identification was not about gender but eroticism." Although published as a peer-reviewed work in a scientific journal, Dreger's paper seemed astonishingly acrimonious, remarking that,

> "trans activists ... have behaved so crazily, the entire population they "represent" has been marked by researchers as being too unstable and dangerous to bother with." [36]

The editor of ASB is Dr. Kenneth Zucker, of the DSM-V Sexual and GID Work Group. Its editorial board includes Dr. Bailey as well as Dr. Ray Blanchard, author of the "autogynephilia" theory and Chair of the DSM-V Paraphilias Subcommittee.[37]

Perhaps the most threatening abuse of scientific authority against dissenting opinion has come from sexologist Dr. Anne Lawrence, also an editorial board member of the *Archives of Sexual Behavior* (ASB), who has strongly supported Blanchard's theories of "autogynephilia." In a commentary article in the ASB, Dr. Lawrence once again repeated personal speculation about sexual orientations of critics of Bailey's book. Moreover, she diagnosed them with "narcissistic disorders." Lawrence invoked a label of "narcissistic rage" to disparage, as further mental illness, the indignation expressed by trans-people in response to psychiatric stereotypes of sexual deviance. She stated,

> "Meanwhile, clinicians and scholars should perhaps be more aware that angry reactions they elicit from nonhomosexual MtF transsexuals might represent narcissistic rage, rather than mature, instrumental anger."[38]

This tactic to discredit dissent by public diagnosis without "client" contact has been termed "medicalization of critics"[39] by psychiatrist Dan Karasic, M.D. of U.C. San Francisco, co-editor of *Sexual and Gender Diagnoses of the Diagnostic and Statistical Manual (DSM): A Reevaluation.*[40]

In an interview for the *New York Times*, Dr. Dreger condemns outrage and dissent from the trans-community with alarming hyperbole, as "problems not only for science but free expression itself."[41] This begs the question, do oppressed people speaking in

109

protest of their own oppression honestly threaten free expression for policy makers? In the discourse of psychiatric policy, who holds the power to bias either scientific enquiry or its dissemination - the authors of the DSM and its allied literature or the subjects of their classification?

At the 1973 annual meeting of the American Psychiatric Association, Dr. Robert Spitzer noted,

> "In the past, homosexuals have been denied civil rights in many areas of life on the ground that because they suffer from a "mental illness" the burden of proof is on them to demonstrate their competence, reliability, or mental stability."[42]

This burden remains as heavy today for gender transcendent people and their supportive clinicians as it was for gay and lesbian people then.

The current diagnostic categories of Gender Identity Disorder and Transvestic Fetishism in the *Diagnostical and Statistical Manual of Mental Disorders* and their supporting literature perpetuate a doctrine of "disordered" gender identity and expression in American psychiatry and psychology. This axiom imposes an unreasonable burden of proof upon gender-variant people who defy this stereotype, upon researchers and scholars who present opposing data, and upon change to the status quo in the DSM. Given harsh consequences that the current diagnoses of mental illness and sexual deviance inflict on human dignity, civil justice and access to medical treatment, should the burden of proof instead be guided by reduction of harm to people? In drafting the Fifth Edition of the DSM, members of Sexual and Gender Identity Disorders Work Group have a fresh opportunity to examine all of the evidence and question the premise that gender identities and expression that differ from birth sex roles are inherently disordered.

[1] I. Reitman and B. Brillstein, directors, *Ghostbusters*, Columbia Pictures, 1984.

[2] B. Alexander, "What's 'normal' sex? Shrinks seek definition," MSNBC, http://www.msnbc.msn.com/id/24664654/ .

[3] Lilienfeld, Lynn and Lorh, eds., *Science and Pseudoscience in Clinical Psychology*, Guildford Press, 2004, p.7.

[4] K. Winters, "Gender Dissonance: Diagnostic Reform of Gender Identity Disorder for Adults," *Sexual and Gender Diagnoses of the Diagnostic and Statistical Manual (DSM): A Reevaluation*, Ed. Dan Karasic, MD. and Jack Drescher, MD., Haworth Press, 2005; co-published in *Journal of Psychology & Human Sexuality*, Vol. 17 issue 3, pp. 71-89, 2005.

[5] American Psychiatric Association, *Diagnostic and Statistical Manual of Mental Disorders, Fourth Edition*, Text Revision, Washington, D.C., 2000, p.577, 580.

[6] Spitzer, First, Gibbon, Williams, eds., *Treatment Companion to the Dsm-IV-TR Casebook*, American Psychiatric Publishing, 2004, pp. 128-134.

[7] A. Speigel, "Two Families Grapple with Sons' Gender Preferences," National Public Radio, *All Things Considered*," http://www.npr.org/templates/story/story.php?storyId=90247842, May 7, 2008.

[8] Trans-Youth Family Allies, www.imatyfa.org.

[9] Personal correspondence, Just Eveln, TYFA Director.

[10] M. Potter, "Second Nature," *5280*, March 2008. http://www.5280.com/issues/story_for_print.php?pageID=1017

[11] K. Zucker and S. Bradley, *Gender Identity Disorder and Psychosexual Problems in Children and Adolescents*, Guilford Press, 1995, pp. 280-282.

[12] K. Drummond, S. Bradley, M. Peterson-Badali, and K. Zucker, "A follow-up study of girls with gender identity disorder," *Developmental Psychology*, v. 44,1, Jan 2008, 34-45.

[13] A. De Vries, T. Steensma, P. Cohen-Kettenis, "Effects of GNRH Analogue Treatment to Delay Puberty: Effects on Psychological Functioning at

16 Years," World Professional Association for Transgender Health, 20th Biennial Symposium, Chicago, Sep 2007.

[14] Cole, C., O'Boyle, M., Emory, L., and Meyer, W (1997), "Comorbidity of Gender Dysphoria and Other Major Psychiatric Diagnoses," Archives of Sexual Behavior, Vol. 26, No. 1, Feb. 1997, p.25.

[15] E. Hooker, "A Preliminary Analysis of Group Behavior of Homosexuals." *Journal of Psychology*, #41, p. 219, 1956

[16] C. Mate-Kole, M. Freschi , and A. Robin, "A controlled study of psychological and social change after surgical gender reassignment in selected male transsexuals." *Brit J Psychiat, v.* 157: pp. 261-264, 1990.

[17] F. Pfäfflin, A. Junge , *Sex Reassignment: Thirty Years of International Follow-Up Studies after SRS — A Comprehensive Review, 1961-1991.* 1992, English translation 1998. http://209.143.139.183/ijtbooks/pfaefflin/1000.asp

[18] J. Morris, *Conundrum: An Extraordinary Narrative of Transsexualism*, Holt, 1987.

[19] J. Green, *Becoming a Visible Man*, Vanderbilt University Press, 2004

[20] D. McCloskey, *Crossing: A Memoir*, University of Chicago Press, 1999.

[21] Kailey, *Just Add Hormones: An Insider's Guide to the Transsexual Experience*, Beacon, 2006.

[22] L. Conway, "Transsexual Women's Successes: Links and Photos," http://ai.eecs.umich.edu/people/conway/TSsuccesses/TSsuccesses.html ; "Successful TransMen: Links and Photos," http://ai.eecs.umich.edu/people/conway/TSsuccesses/TransMen.html.; Professor Conway's own extraordinary narrative is available at www.lynnconway.com.

[23] K. Winters (under pen-name K. Wilson), "The Disparate Classification of Gender and Sexual Orientation in American Psychiatry," 1998 Annual Meeting of the American Psychiatric Association, Workshop IW57, Transgender Issues, Toronto, Ontario Canada, June 1998. This paper is a revised and expanded version of a previous article of the same title, published in *Psychiatry On-Line, The International Forum for Psychiatry*, Priory Lodge Education, Ltd., April, 1997, www.priory.com/psych/disparat.htm.

24 P. Burke, *Gender Shock, Exploding the Myths of Male and Female*, Anchor Books, 1996, p. 100.

25 S. Wilkinson, "Drop the Barbie! If You Bend Gender Far Enough, Does It Break?" *Brain, Child*, fall 2001, http://www.brainchildmag.com/essays/fall2001_wilkinson.htm

26 R. Isay, "Remove Gender Identity Disorder in DSM," *Psychiatric News*, v. 32,9, p. 13, November 1997.

27 K. Zucker, "Gender Identity Disorder in the DSM-IV"[Letter to the Editor], *J Sex and Marital Therapy*, vol 25, 1999, pp. 5-9.

28 F. Olyslager and L.Conway, "On the Calculation of the Prevalence of Transsexualism," WPATH 20th International Symposium, Chicago, Illinois, 2007. http://ai.eecs.umich.edu/people/conway/TS/Prevalence/Reports/Prevalence %20of%20Transsexualism.pdf , Submitted for publication, *International Journal of Transgenderism* (IJT).

29 M. Horton, "The Cost of Transgender Health Benefits," Out and Equal Convention, Denver CO, 2006, http://www.tgender.net/taw/thbcost.html

30 American Psychological Association, "Report of the Task Force on Gender Identity and Gender Variance," p. 37, www.apa.org/pi/lgbc/transgender/2008TaskForceReport.pdf

31 J. Bailey, *The Man Who Would Be Queen: The Science of Gender-Bending and Transsexualism*, Joseph Henry Press, 2003.

32 R. Blanchard, "The Classification and Labeling of Nonhomosexual Gender Dysphorias," Archives of Sexual Behavior, Vol 18⁴, Aug 1989, pp. 315-334.

33 B. Allison, "Janice Raymond and Autogynephilia," 2004 http://www.drbecky.com/raymond.html

34 M. Wyndzen, "Autogynephilia and Ray Blanchard's mis-directed sex-drive model of transsexuality," 2003, http://www.genderpsychology.org/autogynephilia/ray_blanchard/

[35] J. Bailey, K. Triea, "What Many Transgender Activists Don't Want You to Know and Why You Should Know It Anyway," *Perspectives in Biology and Medicine*, v. 50, 4, autumn 2007, pp. 527-529, 531.

[36] A. Dreger, "The Controversy Surrounding The Man Who Would Be Queen: A Case History of the Politics of Science, Identity, and Sex in the Internet Age," *Arch Sex Behav*, v. 37, 2008, p. 387, 413, http://bioethics.northwestern.edu/faculty/work/dreger/controversy_tmwwb q.pdf

[37] *Archives of Sexual Behavior, The Official Publication of the International Academy of Sex Research*, Editorial Board, http://www.springer.com/public+health/journal/10508?detailsPage=editorial Board

[38] A. Lawrence, "Shame and Narcissistic Rage in Autogynephilic Transsexualism," *Arch Sex Behav* , v. 37, p. 457.

[39] D. Karasic, "Sexuality and Gender Identity in the DSM V: Current Controversies," UCSF Grand Rounds in the Dept of Psychiatry, U.C. San Francisco, June 26, 2008.

[40] D. Karasic and J. Drescher, Eds., *Sexual and Gender Diagnoses of the Diagnostic and Statistical Manual (DSM) a Reevaluation*, Haworth Press, 2005

[41] B. Carey, "Criticism of a Gender Theory, and a Scientist Under Siege," *The New York Times*, August 21, 2007

[42] R. Spitzer, "A Proposal About Homosexuality and the APA Nomenclature: Homosexuality as an Irregular Form of Sexual Behavior and Sexual Orientation Disturbance as a Psychiatric Disorder," *American Journal of Psychiatry*, Vol. 130, No. 11, November 1973 p.1216

[43] E. Hendrick, "Quiet Down There! The Discourse of Academic Freedom as Defence of Hierarchy in the Aftermath of J. Michael Bailey's The Man Who Would Be Queen," panel presentation, 2008 National Women's Studies Association conference, June 21, 2008. http://ai.eecs.umich.edu/people/conway/TS/News/US/NWSA/Papers/Qui et_Down_There.pdf

A preliminary revision of this essay was posted at GID Reform Advocates: K. Winters, "Blinded Me with Science: The Burden of Proof" October 20, 2008, www.gidreform.org/blog2008Oct20.html

Autogynephilia and *Homosexual* Gender Dysphoria

In the Third Edition of the *Diagnostic and Statistical Manual of Mental Disorders* (DSM) in 1980, the American Psychiatric Association explained the reasons for removing the diagnostic category of homosexuality:[1]

> "The crucial issue in determining whether or not homosexuality per se should be regarded as a mental disorder is not the etiology of the condition, but its consequences and the definition of mental disorder." [2]

This marked a significant shift in diagnostic policy toward the consequence of a condition rather than speculation of its cause. Two decades later, the APA discarded this principle by emphasizing the controversial and inflammatory theory of "autogynephilia" in the supporting text of Gender Identity Disorder diagnosis of the DSM-IV-TR:

> "Adult males who are sexually attracted to females, to both males and females, or to neither sex usually report a history of erotic arousal associated with the thought or image of oneself as a woman (termed autogynephilia)."[3]

This statement and its supporting literature, that hypothesize sexual deviance as a cause of transsexualism, have sparked dissent among clinicians and researchers and outrage within the trans-community.[4-8] While theories around "autogynephilia" seem exceptionally impervious to contrary evidence, the controversy has raised questions about tolerance and bias in American

117

Psychiatry- at what point do bad stereotypes preclude good science?

The term "autogynephilia," meaning "love of oneself as a woman," was first introduced by Dr. Raymond Blanchard of the Clarke Institute of Psychiatry, now known as the Centre for Addiction and Mental Health in Toronto. He is currently chairman of the Paraphilias Subcommittee for the upcoming DSM-V. Blanchard stated that,

> "All gender dysphoric males who are not sexually oriented toward men are instead sexually oriented toward the thought or image of themselves as women."[9]

The absolutism in this statement, in the words "all" and "instead," seems astonishing.[10] It reduces a broad diversity of sexuality among transwomen to two narrow maligning stereotypes: either "homosexual males" in denial of a "homosexual" identity or pathological narcissistic "males" sexually attracted to themselves. This strict dichotomy stands in contrast to the words of Dr. Alfred Kinsey, the father of modern sexology:

> "The world is not divided into sheeps and goats. Not all things are black nor all things white. It is a fundamental of taxonomy that nature rarely deals with discrete categories. Only the human mind invents categories and tries to force facts into separated pigeon-holes. The living world is a continuum in each and every one of its aspects. The sooner we learn this concerning sexual behavior the sooner we shall reach a sound understanding of the realities of sex."[11]

Although the phenomenon described by "autogynephilia," arousal to thoughts of being women, appears in personal narratives by some transwomen,[12] there is no apparent basis for projecting this stereotype upon all lesbian, bisexual and asexual transwomen. Dr. Blanchard conflates association with causation by using the phrase "erotic arousal in association with the thought or image of themselves as women" interchangeably with "erotically aroused by the thought or image..."[13] However, "association with" is not the same as "aroused by."

What role do natal or birth-assigned women play in their own sexual fantasies? No one would consider it odd or "fetishistic" for non-transwomen to be themselves on the stage of their sex lives. Nor would anyone assume that they are aroused by their self-image as women rather than by their partners. Why then are lesbian and bisexual transwomen treated so differently by American psychiatry and psychology? For transwomen born without female anatomy, incongruence of their bodies with self-identities pose understandable barriers to sexual expression.

The desire to remove these barriers is perhaps more accurately described as an adaptive accommodation to a physiological deficiency. Does the image of a female body "interfere" with normal attractions as Blanchard suggests[14] or does it enable them?

Dr. Blanchard's studies of clinical patients reporting "erotic arousal in association with cross-dressing" were presented as "fetishistic cases."[15-16] His findings have been criticized by psychologist and community advocate Dr. Madeline Wyndzen as having never been replicated, excluding control groups of birth-assigned women, and for inferring causation from mere observational data.[17] For gender dysphoric youth with no access to medical transition procedures, is cross-dressing a "fetishistic" pathology, or is it an adaptive coping strategy to an incongruent

119

body? It seems more plausible that cross-dressing represents an accommodation to conceal or disguise anatomy which poses barriers to lesbian or bisexual expression or fantasy.

Dr. Blanchard's studies omitted control groups of birth-assigned women and overlooked the roles that fashion, clothing and lingerie play in their sexual expression and fantasy. For birth-assigned women, sexual expression is accompanied by a $300 billion fashion industry in the U.S.[18] but without diagnosis of fetishistism or pathology. Dr. Sigmund Freud, however, noted how fashion accompanies sexuality with a metaphorical remark:

> "In the world of everyday experience, we can observe that half of humanity must be classed among the clothes fetishists. All women, that is, are clothes fetishists. ... For them clothes take the place of parts of the body, and to wear the same clothes means only to be able to show what the others can show, means only that one can find in her everything that one can expect from women, an assurance which the woman can give only in this form."[19]

Freud's observations on the role of clothing in the expression of womanhood seem relevant to Blanchard's presumption of "autogynephilic" pathology in transwomen, for whom "clothes take the place of parts of the body" - parts that nature did not provide.

What of transwomen who attest attraction to women and frequently are in very long-term relationships, partnerships and marriages with women? Blanchard's theory of "autogynephilia," like Dr. Magnus Hirschfeld's "automonosexualism,"[20] implies that all transwomen not exclusively attracted to men are incapable of genuine attraction to other women.[21] However, historical clinical literature reports 20 to 30 percent of transsexual women attracted primarily or exclusively to other women.[22-23] These early figures are likely understated, as attraction to women posed barriers to access to hormonal and surgical transition care. Nonclinical surveys report higher rates of same-sex orientation (with regard to affirmed identity, not assigned birth sex).[24-25] It seems paradoxical that these women are labeled as "autogynephiles" on the basis of their attraction to women, while that very label contradicts the validity of their attraction to women.

How does the "autogynephilia" hypothesis, that "all" transwomen are attracted to men or "instead" to themselves, explain the existence of long-term relationships with other women? In Colorado, writer Laurie Cicotello's story of her remarkable family is a profound counterexample.

In 1997, Ms. Cicotello testified before the Colorado legislature with her father, Dana, a transwoman, educator and advocate respected throughout the transgender community. They spoke in opposition to an anti-gay and lesbian marriage bill that would have threatened her parents' legal same-sex marriage of forty years at the time of this writing. Laurie described how she stood with her parents later that year, hands clasped together over their heads, before fifty-five thousand people at the Denver PrideFest Rally. In a state known in the 90s for religious intolerance of GLBT diversity, Dana proclaimed to the crowd, "I've got your family values, right here!"[26]

Theories of "autogynephilia" not only associate hurtful stereotypes of sexual deviance with transwomen, they presume "erotic anomalies" to be the cause of gender dysphoria and the motivation for transition. Speaking of lesbian, bisexual and asexual transwomen not primarily attracted to men, Dr. Blanchard states:

"This hypothesis asserts that the various discriminable syndromes of non-homosexual gender dysphoria are the results of autogynephilia interacting with additional constitutional or experiential factors."[27]

Bailey and Triea recently reiterated this view that "nonhomosexual transsexuals experience erotic arousal at the idea of becoming a woman, and this arousal motivates them to become women."[28] However, neither they nor Blanchard offered evidence of a causal relationship between a sexual affinity for one's-self and gender dysphoria (intense distress with one's assigned birth sex or natal anatomy.)

This body of theory seems to proffer the circular reasoning that:

If "autogynephilia" is associated with all lesbian and bisexual transsexual women, then it must be the cause of gender dysphoria for them.

And—

If "autogynephilia" is the cause of gender dysphoria in lesbian and bisexual transsexual women, then all of them must be "autogynephilic."

Proponents of these stereotypes of sexual deviance do not ask the fundamental questions about how gender identity forms in all human beings, transgender and cisgender. They neglect to include control groups of birth-assigned women with their limited, clinical samples of transwomen. They most often neglect to include nonclinical samples of transitioned women living full lives in the real world. They fail to consider the similarities between birth-assigned women and transitioned women of all sexual orientations, similarities so profound that the existence of large numbers of transitioned women remains unacknowledged by psychiatric researchers.[29] Moreover, the proven efficacy of social and medical transition in relieving the distress of gender dysphoria and improving quality of lives[30-31] remains unexplained by "autogynephilic" theories of etiology.

The corollary of "autogynephilia" theory postulates that straight transwomen attracted to men do not possess female gender identities but are merely gay men in denial. They are branded by Blanchard with a maligning label of "homosexual male transsexuals."[32] He asserts that straight and lesbian/bisexual/asexual transwomen are so fundamentally different that they represent two entirely distinct "disorders,"

> "The feminine gender identity that develops in homosexual males is different from the feminine gender identity that develops in heterosexual males. In other words, homosexual and heterosexual men cannot "catch" the same gender identity disorder in the way that homosexual and heterosexual men can both "catch" the identical strain of influenza virus. Each class of men is susceptible to its own type of gender identity disorder and only its own type of gender identity disorder."[33]

Dr. Blanchard's certainty of mutually exclusive transsexual types based on sexual orientation seems peculiar within sexology, where both gender identity[34] and sexual orientation[11] have long been viewed as continuous rather than dichotomous. He bases this assumption on differences in "a history of erotic arousal in association with cross-dressing," in ages of presentation for "professional help," and in "degrees of childhood femininity" within clinical populations. Correlating these attributes to the lack or presence of attraction to males, Blanchard concludes that "the main varieties of nonhomosexual gender dysphoria are more similar to each other than any of them is to the homosexual type."[35]

However, a recent study of gender-dysphoric MTF subjects reported no significant difference in scores on a gender identity/gender dysphoria questionnaire with regard to sexual orientation.[36] This result was not explained by Blanchard's assumption of fundamentally different gender identities.

Blanchard's analogy of gender-variant identities to communicable disease is offensive. His research does not consider the shame and guilt that force gender dysphoric youth and adults into the closet, often suffering for decades. For example, "degrees of childhood femininity" may indicate degrees of closeted self-expression far more than innate femininity. The doctrine of "autogynephilic" dichotomy neglects different social pressures faced by gender dysphoric youth and adults, based on their sexual orientations. These differences in social oppression would certainly impact their ability to emerge from the closet and express their inner identities.

Inferring gender identity based on age of clinical presentation is especially troubling, given Zucker and Bradley's observation that gender-variant youth are "invariably" referred by adults and not by themselves.[37] Admission to clinics that practice gender-reparative therapy (attempting to change one's gender identity or expression) may well indicate parental intolerance rather than gender identity per se. For MTF youth, dates of clinical presentation may likely signify the dates they were caught by their parents in their sisters' clothes and little more. For any closeted population, it is wrong to confuse "onset" with presentation to a mental institution or clinic.

For straight transwomen attracted to men, Dr. Blanchard states that all "homosexual gender dysphorics are sufficiently similar to be treated as one diagnostic group."[38] The statement introduces "homosexual gender dysphorics" as a term of mental disorder. However the theory that attraction to men is the sole motivation for transition does not explain why the vast majority of gay males do not transition. It does not explain very low rates of surgical regrets for transwomen, with and without partners or spouses. Nor does it explain very young children who are painfully distressed with their assigned birth sex or why some transition years before adolescence. What then would differentiate straight transwomen and girls from gay males, if gender dysphoria is hypothesized to exclude any innate sense of gender identity?

Perhaps the model of "homosexual gender dysphoria" assumes that living as transsexual women is somehow socially advantageous to living as gay men. To the contrary, gay men possess greater social status, economic privilege and civil rights protection than transwomen in the U.S. and much of the world. For example, 20 states currently prohibit workplace discrimination based on sexual orientation, while only 12 include protection based on gender identity. 88 percent of U.S. Fortune 500 employers prohibit discrimination based on sexual orientation versus 25 percent that include gender identity.[39] It seems farfetched that "all" straight transwomen who forfeit social status to transition would be driven only by attraction to men.

[1] Diagnostic nomenclature of homosexuality was actually removed from the DSM in intermediate stages over a fourteen year span. Homosexuality per se was replaced by Sexual Orientation Disturbance in the seventh printing of the DSM-I in 1973 and by Ego-Dystonic Homosexuality in the DSM-III in 1980. This was removed from the DSM-III-R in 1987. While APA policy now affirms that same sex orientation is no longer regarded as mental disorder, two diagnostic categories remain in the current DSM-IV-TR that may be used to diagnose homosexuality as mental illness: Sexual Disorder Not Otherwise Specified and Gender Identity Disorder of Children.

[2] American Psychiatric Association, Diagnostic *and Statistical Manual of Mental Disorders*, Third Edition, 1980 p. 380.

[3] American Psychiatric Association, *Diagnostic and Statistical Manual of Mental Disorders*, Fourth Edition, Text Revision, Washington, D.C., 2000, p. 578.

[4] H. Cassell, "Controversy Dogs Sexuality Researcher," Bay Area Reporter, October 4 2007, http://ebar.com/news/article.php?sec=news&article=2274

[5] M. Wyndzen, "Everything You Never Wanted to Know About Autogynephilia (But Were Afraid You Had To Ask)," Psychology of Gender Identity & Transgenderism, 2004, http://www.genderpsychology.org/autogynephilia/

[6] A. Dreger, "The Controversy Surrounding The Man Who Would Be Queen: A Case History of the Politics of Science, Identity, and Sex in the Internet Age," *Archives of Sexual Behavior*, Vol. 37, No. 3, June 2008, pp. 366-421. http://www.bioethics.northwestern.edu/faculty/work/dreger/controversy_t mwwbq.pdf

[7] L. Conway, "An investigation into the publication of J. Michael Bailey's The Man Who Would Be Queen," 2004, http://ai.eecs.umich.edu/people/conway/TS/LynnsReviewOfBaileysBook.ht ml

[8] A. James, "'Autogynephilia': A disputed diagnosis," Transsexual Road Map, 2004, http://www.tsroadmap.com/info/autogynephilia.html

[9] R. Blanchard, "The Classification and Labeling of Nonhomosexual Gender Dysphoria," *Archives of Sexual Behavior*, v. 18 n. 4, 1989, p. 322-323.

[10] K. Wilson (former pen-name for Kelley Winters), "Autogynephilia: New Medical Thinking or Old Stereotype?" *Transgender Forum Magazine*, April 16, 2000. http://www.gidreform.org/kwauto00.html

[11] A. Kinsey, W. Pomeroy, and C.Martin. *Sexual Behavior in the Human* Male, W.B. Saunders: 1948, p. 639.

[12] A. Lawrence, "28 narratives about autogynephilia," 2004, http://www.annelawrence.com/agnarratives.html.

[13] R. Blanchard, "Early History of the Concept of Autogynephilia," *Archives of Sexual Behavior*, Vol. 34, No. 4, August 2005, p. 439.

[14] Blanchard 1989, p. 323.

[15] R. Blanchard, "Typology of male-to-female transsexualism," *Archives of Sexual Behavior*, v. 14, 1985, pp. 247-261.

[16] R. Blanchard, "Nonhomosexual Gender Dysphoria," *Archives of Sexual Behavior*, v. 24, 1988, pp. 188-193.

[17] Wyndzen M.H. (2004). "A Personal and Scientific look at a Mental Illness Model of Transgenderism," *Division 33 Newsletter*, Society for the Psychological Study of Lesbian, Gay, and Bisexual Issues, Vol. 20, No. 1, Spring. P.3. http://www.genderpsychology.org/autogynephilia/apa_div_44.html

[18] C. Horyn, "Fashion Industry Rallies to Aid Designer in Trouble, New York Times, May 7, 2007.

[18] A. Hamlyn, "Freud, Fabric, Fetish," *Textile: The Journal of Cloth and Culture*, Volume 1, Number 1, 1 March 2003 , pp. 8-26.

[20] Blanchard 1989, p. 317.

[21] Wilson 2000.

[22] J. Wålinder, *Transsexualism: A Study of Forty-Three Cases*, Scandinavian University Books, 1967.

23 K. Freund, B. Steiner, & S. Chan, "Two Types of Cross-Gender Identity," *Arch. Sex Beh* 11: 49-63.

24 J. Xavier, "The Washington Transgender Needs Assessment Survey," US Helping Us – People Into Living, Inc., Washington D.C., 2000, http://www.glaa.org/archive/2000/tgneedsassessment1112.shtml

25 P. De Sutter, K. Kira, A. Verschoor and A. Hotimsky, "The Desire to have Children and the Preservation of Fertility in Transsexual Women: A Survey," *International Journal of Transgenderism*, v. 6 n. 3, 2002, http://www.symposion.com/ijt/ijtvo06no03_02.htm

26 L. Cicotello, "She'll Always be my Daddy," in N. Howey and E. Samuels, *Out of the Ordinary: Essays on Growing Up with Gay, Lesbian, and Transgender Parents*, Macmillan 2000, pp. 131-142.

27 Blanchard 1989, p. 232.

28 J. Bailey, K. Triea, "What Many Transgender Activists Don't Want You to Know and Why You Should Know It Anyway," *Perspectives in Biology and Medicine*, v. 50, 4, autumn 2007, pp. 527-529, 531.

29 F. Olyslager and L.Conway, "On the Calculation of the Prevalence of Transsexualism," WPATH 20th International Symposium, Chicago, Illinois, 2007. http://ai.eecs.umich.edu/people/conway/TS/Prevalence/Reports/Prevalence%20of%20Transsexualism.pdf , Submitted for publication, *International Journal of Transgenderism* (IJT).

30 F. Pfäfflin, A. Junge , *Sex Reassignment: Thirty Years of International Follow-Up Studies after SRS — A Comprehensive Review, 1961-1991.* 1992, English translation 1998. http://209.143.139.183/ijtbooks/pfaefflin/1000.asp

31 A. Lawrence, "Factors associated with satisfaction or regret following male-to-female sex reassignment surgery," Archives of Sexual Behavior, v. 32 n. 4, August 2003, pp. 299-315, http://www.accessmylibrary.com/coms2/summary_0286-23760688_ITM

32 Blanchard 1985, p. 247.

33 Blanchard 2005, p. 443.

[34] Benjamin, H. (1966). The transsexual phenomenon. New York: The Julian Press, page 22-23.

[35] Blanchard 1989, pp. 315, 324-325.

[36] J. Deogracias, L. Johnson, H. Meyer-Bahlburg, S. Kessler, J. Schober, K. Zucker, "The gender identity/gender dysphoria questionnaire for adolescents and adults," *Journal of Sex Research*, v. 44 n. 4, November 2007, pp. 370-379, http://findarticles.com/p/articles/mi_m2372/is_4_44/ai_n27467813***

[37] K. Zucker and S. Bradley, "Gender Identity Disorder and Transvestic Fetishism," in S. Netherton, D. Holmes and C. Walker, eds, *Child and Adolescent Psychological Disorders: A Comprehensive Textbook*, Oxford Univ Press, 1999, p. 386.

[38] Blanchard 1989, p. 331.

[39] Human Rights Campaign, Inc., *The State of the Work Place 2006-2007*, http://www.hrc.org/documents/State_of_the_Workplace.pdf

A preliminary revision of this essay was posted at GID Reform Advocates: K. Winters, "Blinded Me with Science: The Infallible Derogatory Hypothesis, Part 1" November 10, 2008, www.gidreform.org/blog2008Nov10.html

The Infallible Derogatory Hypotheses

Dr. Ray Blanchard's taxonomy of "autogynephilia" and "homosexual transsexualism" followed a long tradition of dividing transsexual women into categorical buckets based on sexual orientation. This view ignored co-occurring human diversity of sexual orientation and gender identity and held that male-to-female transsexualism was a phenomenon of effeminate male homosexuality, while the label of "transvestism" was associated with heterosexual men. Hence, diagnostic nomenclature and research literature have for decades favored candidates for surgical transition care who would have heterosexual outcomes (i.e., transwomen attracted to men).[1]

In the 1960s, Dr. Harry Benjamin's defined two types of so-called "true transsexuals" as distinct from "transvestites" and "non-surgical transsexuals," based on Kinsey's scale of sexual orientation. Those attracted to men were labeled "high intensity," resembling Blanchard's "homosexual" label. Benjamin described asexual, "auto-erotic" and some bisexual individuals as "low intensity" or "nonsurgical transsexual." He labeled transsexual women attracted to women mostly as "transvestites,"[2] and the belief that those termed "transvestites" were not gender dysphoric or attracted to men held until the 1980s.

While Benjamin emphasized that his six types of MTF transsexualism "are not and never can be sharply separated," psychiatrist Robert Stoller insisted on exclusive division of transsexualism from "transvestism." Stoller considered a single episode of cross-dressing *associated* with sexual arousal sufficient to exclude a diagnosis of transsexualism[3] and therefore denial of access to transition medical care. (Like Blanchard today, Stoller conflated "association" with erotic causation in his literature.) This view was reflected in the DSM-III-R,[4] where concurrent diagnosis of Transvestic Fetishism and GID of Adolescence or Adulthood, Nontranssexual Type (GIDAANT) or Transsexualism were not allowed[5].

In the real world, however, large numbers of transsexual women, who were attracted to women and applied for corrective transition surgeries, refuted the theory that presumed them to be gay men. They were called such uncomplimentary names as "transvestic transsexuals,"[6] "aging transvestites"[7] and "non-transsexual men applying for SRS."[8] Where researchers in other scientific disciplines might have questioned the premise in view of contrary data, psychiatric researchers leapt to an incredible assumption: that there must be an additional independent "etiology" or cause for MTF transsexualism. Early on, this second "etiology" was described as a "regression" of transvestism into transsexualism, inexplicably "provoked" by stress.[9] In the late 1970s, Person and Ovesey offered a Hitchcockian psychoanalytic explanation of this process:

> "At times of stress, ... transvestites frantically step up the pace of acting out. Should such reparative measures fail, they regressively fall back on the more primitive fantasy of symbiotic fusion with the mother. It is at this point that transsexual impulses break out and may go on to full-blown transsexual syndrome (secondary transsexualism)."[10]

Blanchard's theory of "autogynephilia" emerged later to fill this role. Deogracias, et al., recently proposed that the similarity of transwomen, regardless of sexual orientation, supports a "concept of equifinality," meaning that the same effect or end state can result from completely different causes.[11]

I am very skeptical of this conclusion, as data that contradict a hypothesis most likely call the validity of the hypothesis into question. Those of us in the physical sciences and engineering often use the principle of Occam's Razor to discern credible from unlikely theories. Contrary to the notion of equifinality, it asserts that simpler parsimonious theories are more likely to be true than twisted complex theories, if all other considerations are equal.

Is it credible that the same effect, gender dysphoria, comes from not one but two unrelated causes depending upon the sexual orientation of the person? Is this science, or do these proliferating theories represent a defensive response - a denial of contradicting evidence that challenges the status-quo? Perhaps Occam's Razor would be good medicine for the behavioral sciences as well.[12]

Moreover, a corner-stone of scientific methodology is the falsifiability of hypotheses -- the possibility that a hypothesis may be refuted by evidence or experiment. Theories are widely considered to be scientific only if they are falsifiable. By capriciously spawning a new independent theory of "autogynephilia" to explain the existence of transwomen who were not exclusively attracted to men, these researchers rendered the original hypothesis of "homosexual male" transsexualism to be unfalsifiable.

In my view, this does not suggest equifinality. Rather, it is evidence of a dubious hypothesis that conveniently metastasizes in the face of contradicting data. It is evidence that the development of gender identity in all people, trans and cisgender alike, is not yet understood.

In recent years, Dr. Blanchard has attempted to draw a distinction between "autogynephilia" as a sexual phenomenon from the other meanings associated with the term, including his own controversial theories.[13] However, the word "autogynephilia" has evolved far beyond sexual taxonomy and theoretical speculation to carry a derogatory context of its own. It has become an offensive epithet to many transwomen. For example, Blanchard and collaborators have grouped "autogynephilia" (lesbian, bisexual and asexual transwomen) with pedophilia, fetishism and even apotemnophilia (desire for limb amputation).[14-15] This reinforces some of the most stigmatizing and dehumanizing false stereotypes that transsexual women bear in society.

In addition, the terms "autogynephilia" and "homosexual transsexual" are now associated with extremely offensive remarks and stereotypes about transsexual and other transgender women. Here are but a few quotes from a very controversial book by Dr. J. Michael Bailey of Northwestern University, entitled *The Man Who Would Be Queen: The Science of Gender-Bending and Transsexualism.*[16]

- "The Man Who Would be Queen" - this maligning description of transsexual women in the book title is accompanied by a cover photo that offensively caricatures them.
- "The autogynephile's main romantic target is herself." – implying that transsexual women not exclusively attracted to men are not capable of attraction to women.
- "Autogynephiles do not typically look or act very feminine" - ridiculing transsexual women for not fitting the author's image of what women are "supposed" to look like.

- "Men Trapped in Men's Bodies" – in reference to transsexual women labeled as "autogynephiles," this chapter title is a quote from Dr. Anne Lawrence.[17]
- "but they don't have the wrong body, they are mentally ill." – in reference to transsexual women labeled as "autogynephiles," Bailey quotes his undergraduate students.
- "homosexual transsexuals are a type of gay man." – in reference to straight transsexual women.
- "homosexual transsexuals are used to living on the margins of society"
- "homosexual transsexuals might be especially well-suited to prostitution."

Published in 2003, this book promoted Blanchard's theories in ways that inflamed a firestorm of outrage[18-21] among the transgender community and supportive allies.

Finally, "autogynephilia" has been used in a punitive context to discredit critics of these theories and negative stereotypes. For example, Bailey and Triea associated disagreement with the theory of "autogynephilic" motivation as symptomatic of "autogynephilia:"

> "although most public transsexual activists appear by their histories and presentations to be nonhomosexual MtF transsexuals, they have generally been hostile toward the idea that nonhomosexual transsexualism is associated with, and motivated by, autogynephilia."[22]

The authors went on to name individuals they termed "transsexual activists" and publicly speculated about their private sexualities. Hence, "autogynephilia" has morphed from a term of taxonomy to a political tool to suppress criticism.

135

To summarize, the term "autogynephilia" means far more than a description of erotic phenomenon. "Autogynephilia," and its corollary "homosexual transsexualism," have come to represent an over-arching body of derogatory stereotypes that are promoted as science but remain dogmatically resilient to contrary evidence:

- "Homosexual transsexual" maligns *all* straight transwomen attracted only to men as "homosexual men."
- "Homosexual transsexual" implies that *all* straight transwomen were motivated to transition by their so-called "homosexuality" or denial of it.
- "Autogynephilia" maligns *all* lesbian and bi transwomen, who are not exclusively attracted to men, as pathologically narcissistic "men."
- "Autogynephilia" insists that *all* lesbian and bi transwomen are attracted to themselves instead of other women, which demeans and undermines these relationships and families.
- "Autogynephilia" implies that *all* lesbian and bi transwomen are motivated to transition primarily by sexual paraphilia or deviance, undermining their legitimacy and dignity as women.
- "Autogynephilia" denies that transwomen who live happy and full lives as women, regardless of sexual orientation, possess any inner feminine gender identity or "essence."
- "Autogynephilia" is a politically punitive label for transwomen who criticize psychiatric policies and stereotypes.
- "Autogynephilia" is indelibly associated with cruel dehumanizing epithets of transwomen, such as "man who would be queen," and "men trapped in men's bodies."

The term "autogynephilia" has grown to represent an affront to the human dignity and legitimacy of many transitioned women. It serves no constructive purpose in an evidence-based diagnostic nosology. I strongly urge the American Psychiatric Association to remove this offensive term from the supporting text of the GID diagnosis and refrain from adding it to the nomenclature of paraphilias in the DSM-V.

[1] K. Winters (published under pen-name Katherine Wilson) and B. Hammond, "Myth, Stereotype, and Cross-Gender Identity in the DSM-IV," Association for Women in Psychology 21st Annual Feminist Psychology Conference, Portland OR, 1996, http://www.gidreform.org/kwawp96.html.

[2] H. Benjamin, *The transsexual phenomenon*, Julian Press, pp. 23-24.

[3] K. Freund, B. Steiner, S. Chan, "Two Types of Cross-Gender Identity," *Archives of Sexual Behavior*, v. 11, n. 1, 1982, p. 55.

[4] American Psychiatric Associatio, *Diagnostic and Statistical Manual of Mental Disorders*, Third Edition, Revised, 1987, pp.76-77,289.

[5] The diagnostic criteria for Transvestic Fetishism excluded diagnosis of Transsexualism or GIDAANT, and the criteria for GIDAANT excluded erotically motivated cross-dressing and Transvestic Fetishism. The criteria for Transsexualism did not explicitly exclude TF, but were assumed to do so. See Bradley, S., et al. (1991). "Interim Report of the DSM-IV Subcommittee on Gender Identity Disorders," *Archives of Sexual Behavior*, Vol. 20, 1991, No. 4, p.338.

[6] E. Person and L. Ovesey, "The Transsexual Syndrome in Males. II. Secondary Transsexualism," *American Journal of Psychotherapy*, v. 28, pp. 174-193.

[7] T. Wise and J. Meyer, "The Border Area Between Transvestism and Gender Dysphoria: Transvestic Applicants for Sex Reassignment," *Archives of Sexual Behavior*, v. 9 n. 4, 1980, p. 329.

[8] R. Stoller "Gender Identity," in A. Freedman, H. Kaplan, & B. Sadock (eds.), *Comprehensive Textbook of Psychiatry*, 2nd ed., vol II, Williams and Wilkins, pp. 1400-1408.

[9] Wise & Meyer, 1980, p. 340.

[10] E. Person and L. Ovesey, "Transvestism: New Perspectives," 1978, in E. Person, *The Sexual Century*, Yale University Press, 1999, p. 167.

[11] J. Deogracias, L. Johnson, H. Meyer-Bahlburg, S. Kessler, J. Schober, K. Zucker, "The gender identity/gender dysphoria questionnaire for adolescents and adults," *Journal of Sex Research*, v. 44 n. 4, November 2007, pp. 370-379, http://findarticles.com/p/articles/mi_m2372/is_4_44/ai_n27467813***

[12] K. Wilson (former pen-name for Kelley Winters), "Autogynephilia: New Medical Thinking or Old Stereotype?" *Transgender Forum Magazine*, April 16, 2000. http://www.gidreform.org/kwauto00.html

[13] R. Blanchard, "Early History of the Concept of Autogynephilia," *Archives of Sexual Behavior*, Vol. 34, No. 4, August 2005, p. 445.

[14] K. Freund, & R. Blanchard, R., "Erotic target location errors in male gender dysphorics, paedophiles, and fetishists," *British Journal of Psychiatry*, 162, 558–563p. 1993, 558.

[15] A. Lawrence, "Clinical and theoretical parallels between desire for limb amputation and gender identity disorder," *Archives of Sexual Behavior*, v. 35, 2006, 263.

[16] J. Bailey, *The Man Who Would Be Queen: The Science of Gender-Bending and Transsexualism,* Joseph Henry Press, 2003, pp. 172, 178, 183-185, 206.

[17] A. Lawrence, "Men Trapped in Men's Bodies: Autogynephilic Eroticism as a Motive for Seeking Sex Reassignment," 16th Harry Benjamin International Gender Dysphoria Association (HBIGDA) Symposium, London, August 1999.

[18] H. Cassell, "Controversy Dogs Sexuality Researcher," Bay Area Reporter, October 4 2007, http://ebar.com/news/article.php?sec=news&article=2274

[19] A. Dreger, "The Controversy Surrounding The Man Who Would Be Queen: A Case History of the Politics of Science, Identity, and Sex in the Internet Age," *Archives of Sexual Behavior*, Vol. 37, No. 3, June 2008, pp. 366-421. http://www.bioethics.northwestern.edu/faculty/work/dreger/controversy_t mwwbq.pdf

[20] L. Conway, "An investigation into the publication of J. Michael Bailey's The Man Who Would Be Queen," 2004, http://ai.eecs.umich.edu/people/conway/TS/LynnsReviewOfBaileysBook.ht ml

[21] A. James, "'Autogynephilia': A disputed diagnosis," Transsexual Road Map, 2004, http://www.tsroadmap.com/info/autogynephilia.html

[22] J. Bailey, K. Triea, "What Many Transgender Activists Don't Want You to Know and Why You Should Know It Anyway," *Perspectives in Biology and Medicine*, v. 50, 4, autumn 2007, pp. 527.

A preliminary revision of this essay was posted at GID Reform Advocates: K. Winters, "Blinded Me with Science: The Infallible Derogatory Hypothesis, Part 2" November 19, 2008, www.gidreform.org/blog2008Nov19.html

Part IV: The Gender Gulag

You lock the door
And throw away the key
There's someone in my head but it's[just] me.

Pink Floyd, "Brain Damage" 1973
(clarified lightly)

"Gender gulag," attributed to R. Wilchins, *Read My Lips: Sexual Subversion and the End of Gender,* Firebrand, 1997, p. 134.

Gender-Reparative Therapies

On May 9th and 23rd, the American Psychiatric Association (APA) issued statements on "GID and the DSM," repeating that,

> "It is important to recognize that the DSM is a diagnostic manual and does not provide treatment recommendations or guidelines."[1]

This was in response to concern from the transgender community and advocates that the current "gender identity disorder" (GID) diagnosis is biased to facilitate gender-conversion therapies. These are punitive psychotherapies attempting to change the gender identities of gender-variant youth and adults, exemplified in a 2008 National Public Radio interview of Dr. Kenneth Zucker (chairman of the DSM-V Sexual and Gender Identity Disorders work group). He described his therapy regimen for a gender-nonconforming child he diagnosed with Gender Identity Disorder:

> "Bradley would no longer be allowed to spend time with girls. He would no longer be allowed to play with girlish toys or pretend that he was a female character. Zucker said that all of these activities were dangerous to a kid with gender identity disorder." [2]

Such harsh shame and punishment, for behaviors which would be ordinary or exemplary for other children assigned female at birth, drew understandable outrage from many affirmed individuals who were forced to grow up in painfully incongruent gender roles.

A recent joint statement from the National Center for Trangender Equality and other leading advocacy organizations echoed broad concern about gender-conversion and sexual-orientation-conversion therapies:

> "It is inconceivable that in the 21st century any credible scientist or medical professional would recommend any discredited treatment that would attempt to change a person's core gender identity or sexual orientation. Such treatments have no empirical basis and are harmful."[3]

However, the APA's denial of any treatment guidance in the *Diagnostic and Statistical Manual of Mental Disorders IV-TR,* (DSM) was repeated frequently[4] and stated bluntly on the APA DSM FAQ page,

> "No information about treatment is included." [5]

However, does repeating a thing often enough make it true? In fact, diagnostic nomenclature and treatment are inseparably intertwined. This is because the efficacy of all drug and psychotherapy treatments are judged according to specific diagnostic criteria listed in the DSM and ICD. For example, it stands to reason that it would be expedient to improve the efficacy and marketability of a psychopharmacological product by tweaking the diagnostic criteria to favor its strengths. In fact, the APA has been criticized on issues of influence by drug manufacturers on the DSM process [6] and now requires disclosure of financial ties to pharmaceutical corporations by members of the DSM-V Task Force.

According to current DSM-IV-TR, youth and adults driven deep in the closet by gender-conversion therapies no longer meet the four diagnostic criteria for GID[7] and are emancipated from diagnosis of mental disorder. On the other hand, affirmed youth and adults who are happy and well adjusted after transition remain diagnosable with GID and suffer stigma of mental illness and sexual deviance for the rest of their lives.[8,9] Children may be diagnosed with GID strictly on the basis of gender nonconformity, without evidence of gender dysphoria or distress with assigned birth sex (criteria A,B; see Appendix A). Adults and adolescents are implicated with "disordered" gender identity so long as they identify with or pass as other than their assigned birth sex or believe that they were "born the wrong sex" (criteria A,B). Furthermore, current GID criteria fail to clarify that clinically significant distress or impairment, the basis for defining mental illness in the DSM, should exclude societal or family prejudice or intolerance (criterion D). Therefore, the DSM can be used to blame transgender victims of discrimination for their own oppression.

While the current GID diagnostic criteria do not explicitly recommend gender-conversion therapy, they are certainly biased to favor that harmful treatment approach and to contradict the legitimacy of transition. This is a major reason the DSM-V is of great importance to the transgender community and supportive mental health care providers.

[1] American Psychiatric Association, "APA STATEMENT ON GID AND THE DSM-V, " http://www.psych.org/MainMenu/Research/DSMIV/DSMV/APAStatements/APAStatementonGIDandTheDSMV.aspx , May 23, 2008,

[2] A. Speigel, "Two Families Grapple with Sons' Gender Preferences," National Public Radio, All Things Considered," http://www.npr.org/templates/story/story.php?storyId=90247842 , May 7, 2008.

[3] National Center for Transgender Equality (NCTE), Transgender Law and Policy Institute (TLPI), Transgender Law Center (TLC), Transgender Youth Family Allies (TYFA), http://www.pamshouseblend.com/upload/Autumn/TransGroupsDSMStatement.pdf , May 28, 2008. (Disclosure, I was involved in the drafting of this statement)

[4] M. Forstein, "Update on the DSM-V Issue," http://quenchzine.blogspot.com/2008/05/update-on-dsm-v-issue.html , May 15, 2008.

[5] American Psychiatric Association, "Frequently Asked Question About DSM," http://www.psych.org/MainMenu/Research/DSMIV/FAQs/WhatistheDSMandwhatisitusedfor.aspx

[6] L. Cosgrove, S. Krimsky, M. Vijayaraghavan, L. Schneider, "Financial Ties between DSM-IV Panel Members and the Pharmaceutical Industry," *Psychotherapy and Psychodynamics*, Vol 75, No 3, http://content.karger.com/ProdukteDB/produkte.asp?Aktion=ShowAbstract&ProduktNr=223864&Ausgabe=231734&ArtikelNr=91772 , 2006.

[7] American Psychiatric Association, *Diagnostic and Statistical Manual of Mental Disorders*, Fourth Edition, Text Revision, 2000, p. 537.

[8] K. Winters, "Issues of GID Diagnosis for Transsexual Women and Men," http://www.gidreform.org/gid30285.html , 2004/2008.

[9] K. Winters, "Issues of Psychiatric Diagnosis for Gender Nonconforming Youth," http://www.gidreform.org/gid3026.html , 2004/2008

A preliminary revision of this essay was posted at GID Reform Advocates: K. Winters, "Beyond Denial: GID Diagnostic Criteria and Gender-Conversion Therapies" June 16, 2008, www.gidreform.org/blog2008Jun16.html

Voices of the Asylum

In 1860, abolitionist and suffrage leader Susan B. Anthony risked arrest to help a battered wife, who had been committed by her husband to an insane asylum for over a year. Mrs. Phoebe Phelps, a school principal and accomplished author, was imprisoned and allowed no contact with her children, friends or family for nonconformity to the submissive role expected of women. It was remarkably easy to incarcerate women of that time with a diagnosis of "delusions" or in later years "hysteria." After her release by writ of habeas corpus, she asked Ms. Anthony to help her flee the grasp of her abusive husband, a Massachusetts Senator. On Christmas night, Anthony took Mrs. Phelps and her daughter by train to New York City and a chance for freedom.

> "...aware of how often her friends of the Underground Railroad had defied the Fugitive Slave Law and hidden and transported fugitive slaves, Susan decided she would do the same for this cultured intelligent woman, a slave to her husband under the law."[1]

A century and a half later, so much and yet so little have changed. Our country has abolished the atrocity of slavery, enacted civil liberties for people of color and just this month elected our first African American President of the United States. Yet, gender-variant Americans are still incarcerated in mental institutions and physically and emotionally assaulted with drugs and "aversion therapies" for failing to comport to the roles of their assigned birth sex.

149

In 1995, Dr. Deidre McCloskey, a renowned professor of economics at the University of Illinois, Chicago, was taken from her home by sheriff's deputies with "a warrant for arrest for mental examination." Dr. McCloskey was a transsexual woman who had come out of the closet to her family prior to social transition. Deidre's sister, a psychologist, held intolerant views of gender diversity and, like Mrs. Phelps' nineteenth-century husband, was easily able to procure a civil commitment to a psychiatric ward.

Dr. McCloskey was incarcerated not once but twice at her sister's insistence. In *Crossing, a Memoir*,[2] McCloskey described the "treatment protocols" for those seized for gender transgression:

> "...the victim has no civil rights, especially if poor and unable to hire a vigorous lawyer; nothing he says is to be credited; no penalty of perjury or civil liability or even court costs attaches to the people initiating the seizure if their testimony proves to be false; and the psychiatrists do everything to avoid the liability from letting the victim free, are cowardly about taking the responsibility to do so and in effect are exempted from liability for the consequences of a false seizure and an unreasonable detention."

Deidre was interrogated by psychiatrists who displayed utter ignorance about gender dysphoria and the transition process. She was labeled as "manic," resulting from "latent homosexuality," decades after the American Psychiatric Association had removed same-sex orientation from the classification of mental illnesses. One psychiatrist demanded, "Are you a homosexual? Do you wish to become one?" When Deidre responded "no," that she was attracted to women, the doctor was incredulous. Reflecting old stereotypes confusing sexual orientation with gender identity, he responded, "Well, then, why are you doing this?"

To regain her freedom, Dr. McCloskey was forced to pay $8000 in legal fees and, astonishingly, was billed $3000 by the hospitals that falsely imprisoned her. She wondered, "What if I were poor?"

Susan Anthony would be disappointed at how little we have progressed.

The extraordinary narrative of Ms. April Ashley, a British transwoman and fashion model, illustrates the cruelty inflicted on gender-variant individuals in mental institutions in the 1950s and beyond. Attempting suicide at eighteen years old, Ashley was rescued by her long hair from the Mersey river and delivered to the Ormskirk Mental Hospital near Liverpool. She agreed to a regimen of gender-reparative therapy at nearby Walton Hospital, intending to change her feminine identity. April's "treatments" included drugging her with ether while doctors exacted, "Why do you want to be a woman?" Later, the interrogations were punctuated with sodium pentathol injections. Ashley was given massive doses of male hormones. Finally, she was placed in a public ward and administered electroconvulsive therapy:

> "These blitzed souls returned from the convulsion chamber like zombies, their eyes blinking and heavily bloodshot, with an attendant supporting them on each side. A few hours later they awoke in their beds with murderous headaches in comparison to which an aspirin overdose is like a day at the seaside. When it comes to medical matters I'm usually very brave but on these occasions was not."

Ashley's treatment illustrated a recurring theme in gender incarceration: obsessed with attempts to change her gender identity, they neglected the depression and despair that led to her original hospitalization. In spite of her abuse, Ms. Ashley persevered to live her truth.

> "'No matter what you do, you'll never be able to change my mind. I said with a knowledge I didn't know I had."[3]

Ashley prevailed as a remarkable pioneer in the trans-community. She was one of the first patients for corrective genital surgery with Dr. Georges Burou in Morocco, and she appeared in *Vogue* and the movie, The *Road to Hong Kong*, starring Bing Crosby and Bob Hope.

Phyllis Burke, author of *Gender Shock: Exploding the Myths of Male and Female,*[4] told the heartbreaking story of Jamie, a transsexual woman who survived fifteen years of hospitalization from age six. "Jamie did not do boy things, and would not lie about it," Burke explains. Admitted in the late 1950s, Jamie was drugged and given numerous electroconvulsive shock treatments (ECTs) over the span of her imprisonment:

> "The treatments never became less painful, and there was nothing more painful than the shock, not even the rapes by the male patients, not even Mother and Father never returning."

At twenty years old, following an extremely painful ECT treatment, Jamie escaped the institution and made her way to San Francisco and transition to an affirmed female life. Jamie asked Ms. Burke to find as many children like her as she could and write about their stories:

"No one is talking about them, … but there are still kids in the hospitals."

Burke noted that attitudes about childhood gender nonconformity within American psychiatry were influenced by Dr. Martha MacDonald and her 1938 study of eight birth-assigned males at Michael Reese Hospital on the South Side of Chicago.[5] In a paper entitled "Criminally Aggressive Behavior in Passive-Effeminate Boys,"[6] MacDonald associated feminine expression with violent aggression. Contrary to this stereotype, she observed that these youth were "model playmates" in the company of girls and she did not clearly distinguish them as perpetrators of violence in the presence of boys or as victims. Nevertheless, MacDonald advocated psychiatric hospitalization of gender-variant youth - a role that her own institution would fill, decades later, in one of the best known and most tragic stories of the gender gulag.

In his seminal autobiography, *The Last Time I Wore a Dress: A Memoir*,[7] Dylan Scholinski recalled high school years incarcerated in a series of mental institutions with a diagnosis of Gender Identity Disorder.[8] The first of these was Michael Reese Hospital, where the fifteen year-old was termed by doctors "an inappropriate female."

"Can you tell me," Scholinski's father had asked at a prior clinic, "why she won't wear a dress?"

At Michael Reese, the award-winning author described being pressed to the floor under the boot of a guard who ordered, "Shut up, you f***ing crazy-ass queer" – a phrase apparently synonymous with a diagnosis of Gender Identity Disorder; being injected with thorazine; being locked in seclusion; being tied to a bed while touched and assaulted by a male patient on the ward.

153

The attending psychiatrist would ask, "Why don't you put on a dress instead of those crummy jeans?"

At Forest Hospital in Des Plaines, Illinois, Scholinski was told that, "if I appeared more feminine I would be better adjusted." This was followed by daily humiliation with "girly lessons" and make-up sessions:

> "If I didn't emerge from my room with foundation, lip gloss, blush, mascara, eyeliner, eye shadow and feathered hair, I lost points. Without points, I couldn't go to the dining room. I couldn't go anywhere. ...
>
> Ever lied to save yourself? ... Ever been so false your own skin is your enemy?"

After three years of incarceration in three institutions at a cost of one million dollars, Scholinski was finally released when insurance benefits ran out. Dylan ultimately triumphed to become an accomplished artist, author and community advocate in Denver, Colorado. He recently founded the Sent(a)Mental Project, A Memorial to GLBTIQ Suicides.[9]

Trey Polesky, a counselor and GID reform advocate[10] received very similar mistreatment at Forest Hospital in 1990. He told how a psychiatrist diagnosed him with Gender Identity Disorder at age 9 and recommended incarceration to "help me become more in touch with my feminine side." In a program of gender-reparative therapy, he was forced to wear pink and purple dresses and skirts, grow out his hair and read teen fashion magazines to learn to behave "like a girl." Trey recalled,

> "I finally learned to fake my way out in order to be released, though the reparative therapy did nothing but

154

shatter my sense of self confidence in who I was. Essentially, they taught me to hate who I was."

Harsh punishment of gender-variant youth occurs in outpatient as well as residential settings. Dr. Arianna Davis today is an advocate for trans and intersex communities and GID reform.

Though born with an intersex condition and expressing a strong female identity at a very early age, she was assigned male and later diagnosed as mentally ill for not comporting to that assignment. Arianna was subjected to a gender-reparative therapy regimen at UCLA in the 1980s:

> "I was subjected to forced testosterone injections and used as a study subject against my wishes. These things happened (under the physical beatings and punishment - recomended by a therapist of a reparative mindset- the urging of my father and the all too eager compliance of UCLA doctors and researchers)."[11]

Dr. Davis' story raises the point, a painful memory to so many of us, of how physical violence from parents of gender-variant children is encouraged by intolerance from the mental health professions – what is called "the sissy-whupping method."[12] I often remark in my own diversity lectures that if it were possible to beat, shame or coerce the gender identity out of a child, I would not exist and my audience would not be having this conversation with me. Playwright Eve Ensler terms this violence toward young transwomen, "They Beat the Girl Out of My Boy... Or So They Tried," in a 2004 Los Angeles production of *The Vagina Monologues*.[13]

In Aldous Huxley's, *Brave New World*, psychiatric aversion therapies were used to condition the lower classes to hate books.[14] In our real world, aversion therapies have long been the cornerstone of reparative therapies intended to "cure" both gender variance and same-sex orientation. However, the American Psychiatric Association issued position statements in 1998 and 2000 opposing these "conversion" treatments that attempt to change sexual orientation:[15]

> "APA recommends that ethical practitioners refrain from attempts to change individuals' sexual orientation, keeping in mind the medical dictum to First, do no harm."

Sadly, the APA never discouraged analogous gender-reparative therapies attempting to change gender identity or suppress gender expression. Indeed, the dictum of "First, do no harm," did not seem to apply to the treatment of gender-variant people within American psychiatry. Nor have the bounds of human compassion and decency, when it came to enforcing conformity to assigned birth sex. For example, Dr. Ron Langevin of the University of Toronto Clarke Institute of Psychiatry (today known as the Centre for Addiction and Mental Health) promoted inhumane aversion treatment of cross-dressing individuals assigned male at birth in his 1983 book, *Sexual Strands: Understanding and Treating Sexual Anomalies in Men.*[16]

Reminiscent of a scene from Anthony Burgess' *A Clockwork Orange*,[17] Langevin described chemical aversion therapy to "cure" cross-dressing,

> "In chemical aversion therapy, the patient is first administered nausea inducing drugs. When he indicates that he feels sick, his favorite female clothes used for crossdressing are presented. He should touch them and look at them as best he can. Then he is overwhelmed by

the need to vomit. The clothes are withdrawn and the procedure repeated several hours later."

Next, he noted the advantages of "electrical aversion" in offering greater "control" over timing. He described the treatment of a patient:

"The conditioning stimuli were pictures of women wearing panties which were followed by the unconditioned stimulus, electric shock. The shock level was set so the patient found it so uncomfortable, he wanted it stopped. In addition to seeing pictures, he was instructed to handle panties and to imagine himself wearing them. After 41 sessions, he said he was no longer troubled by the "fetish" but a month later, it spontaneously recovered."

Finally, Dr. Langevin introduced a newer form of "shame aversion therapy" used on a "transvestite:"

"...the patient was required to crossdress before a disinterested group of men and women who watched him without reaction or comment. ... In this case, shame replaces electric shock ... the patient was evidently experiencing shame. He was in tears as he crossdressed and had a look of anguish on his face. He attempted suicide the following day according to the investigator." [18]

This unconscionable "treatment" brings to mind a quote by Nurse Ratched of Ken Kesey's *One Flew Over the Cuckoo's Nest*. "Aren't you ashamed?" she demanded.[19]

Ashamed of what, though? Where exactly is the shame in being different? Author Dylan Scholinski perhaps says it best:

157

"But I've proven the doctors wrong. I don't feel disgust in myself or in love.

They are the ones who should be ashamed"[20]

Psychiatric incarceration and abuse of gender-variant youth and adults is facilitated by diagnostic nomenclature that equates difference with disease: nonconformity to assigned birth sex with mental disorder and sexual deviance. It is time for the American Psychiatric Association and other mental health organizations to repudiate the practice of gender-reparative therapies, as they have renounced reparative therapies for sexual orientation. It is time for the APA and the mental health professions to extend an apology to all who have been imprisoned or traumatized in the course of these treatments. In drafting the fifth edition of the *Diagnostic and Statistical Manual of Mental Disorder*, it is time for the APA to remove the classification of Transvestic Fetishism and revise that of Gender Identity Disorder to serve constructive rather than destructive purposes. It is time for new diagnostic nomenclature consistent with the medical principle of "First, do no harm."

[1] A. Lutz, *Susan B. Anthony: Rebel, Crusader, Humanitarian*, Zenger, 1959, p90.

[2] D. McCloskey, *Crossing, a Memoir*, University of Chicago Pres, 2000, pp. 98, 107, 117.

[3] D. Fallowell and A. Ashley, *April Ashley's Odyssey*, Jonathan Cape, London, 1982. http://www.antijen.org/Aprilv1/

[4] P. Burke, *Gender Shock: Exploding the Myths of Male and Female*, Anchor, 1996, pp. 75-84.

[5] Burke 1996, pp. 71-74.

[6] M. MacDonald, "Criminally Aggressive Behavior in Passive-Effeminate Boys," *American Journal of Orthopsychiatry*, v.8, 1938, pp. 70-78.

[7] D. Scholinski and J. Adams, *The Last Time I Wore a Dress: A Memoir*, Riverhead, 1997, pp. x, 6, 7, 33, 56, 57, 80, 117. Dylan Scholinski's name was Daphne at the time of publication.

[8] American Psychiatric Association, <u>Diagnostic and Statistical Manual of Mental Disorders</u>, Fourth Edition, Text Revision, Washington, D.C., 2000, pp. 576-582.

[9] D. Scholinski, "Sent(a)Mental Project, A Memorial to GLBTIQ Suicides," http://www.myspace.com/dylanscholinski

[10] T. Polesky, http://www.gidreform.org/advocate.html#trey

[11] Personal correspondence, A. Davis. See also http://www.gidreform.org/advocate.html

[12] Holly, "The Sissy-Whupping Method," *Feministe*, http://www.feministe.us/blog/archives/2008/05/13/7399/

[13] E. Ensler, "They Beat the Girl Out of My Boy... Or So They Tried," performed by Calpernia Addams, *The Vagina Monologues*, V-Day Los Angeles, February 2, 2004, http://www.deepstealth.com/vday/

[14] A. Huxley, *Brave New World*, Harper, 1932, p. 22.

[15] American Psychiatric Association, "Position Statement: Therapies Focused on Attempts to Change Sexual Orientation (Reparative or Conversion Therapies)," 2000,
http://archive.psych.org/edu/other_res/lib_archives/archives/200001.pdf

[16] R. Langevin, *Sexual Strands: Understanding and Treating Sexual Anomalies in Men*, Lawrence Erlbaum Assoc., 1983.

[17] A. Burgess, *A Clockwork Orange*, William Heinemann (UK) 1962.

[18] Langevin 1983, pp. 222, 224, 254.

[19] K. Kesey, *One Flew Over the Cuckoo's Nest*, Signet, 1963, p. 242.

[20] Scholinski 1997, p. 195.

A preliminary revision of this essay was posted at GID Reform Advocates: K. Winters, "The Gender Gulag: Voices of the Asylum" November 26, 2008, www.gidreform.org/blog2008Nov26.html

Ten Specific Issues with the GID Diagnosis

A few years ago, Dr. Frank Kameny, co-founder of the National Gay and Lesbian Task Force and leader in the effort to remove the classification of homosexuality from the *Diagnostic and Statistical Manual of Mental Disorders* (DSM)[1] offered me this advice:

> "People must know with specificity what you are pushing for."

For the gender madness within the current Gender Identity Disorder (GID) diagnosis,[2] the Devil is perhaps in the details. Overarching issues of social stigma and barriers to medical transition procedures are related to specific flaws in the diagnostic criteria (Appendix A), supporting text, title and placement in the manual. The philosopher Jiddu Krishnamurti said,

> "If we can really understand the problem, the answer will come out of it, because the answer is not separate from the problem."[3]

The following list highlights the most egregious of my own concerns with the current GID diagnosis. While far from comprehensive, it is perhaps a starting point for dialogue about how harm reduction of gender nomenclature might be possible in the DSM-V.

1. Lacks clarity on debilitating distress of gender dysphoria that is experienced by some, defined here as clinically

significant distress with physical sex characteristics or ascribed gender role.[4]

The distress of gender dysphoria that necessitates medical intervention is inadequately described in criterion B of the GID diagnosis in the DSM-IV-TR as "discomfort" or "inappropriateness." For youth, this often-debilitating pain is obfuscated in the diagnostic criterion, which emphasizes nonconformity to gender stereotypes of assigned birth sex rather than clinically significant distress. Adolescents and adults who believe they were "born in the wrong sex" meet criterion B on the basis of that belief, even if their gender dysphoria has been relieved by transition or related medical procedures.

2. **Stigma of mental illness upon emotions and expressions that are ordinary or even exemplary for non-transgender children, adolescents and adults.**

Criterion A for Gender Identity Disorder highlights a desire to be treated as, or "frequently passing as," the affirmed gender as pathological. For children, criteria A and B stress ordinary masculine or feminine expression in clothing, play, games, toys, and fantasy as symptoms of mental "disturbance." They enforce rigid archaic gender stereotypes upon children. The supporting text disparages innocent childhood play as disorder, including Barbie dolls, playing house, Batman and "rough-and-tumble" activity, if they violate stereotypes of assigned birth sex. Incredulously, knitting is implicated as a focus of sexual perversion for adult transwomen in the supporting text.

3. Focus of pathology on nonconformity to assigned birth sex in disregard to the definition of mental disorder, which comprises distress and impairment.

Recent revisions of the DSM increasingly target gender identity and expression that differ from natal or assigned birth sex as disordered. The current diagnostic criteria for GID in the DSM-IV-TR are preoccupied with social gender role nonconformity, especially for children. Identification with the "other sex," meaning other than assigned birth sex, is described as symptomatic regardless of satisfaction and happiness with that identification.

4. Contradicts transition and access to hormonal and surgical treatments, which are well proven to relieve distress of gender dysphoria.

Social role transition, living and passing in affirmed gender roles, and desiring congruent anatomic sex characteristics are listed as "manifestation" of mental pathology in criterion A of Gender Identity Disorder. Requests for hormonal or surgical treatment to relieve gender dysphoria are disparaged as "preoccupation" in criterion B and supporting text, rather than medical necessity. Evidence of medical transition treatment, such as breast development for transwomen or chest reconstruction for transmen, are described in a negative context as "associated features and disorders" of mental illness in the supporting text.

5. Encourages gender-conversion therapies, intended to change or shame one's gender identity or expression.

The DSM is intended as a diagnostic guide without specific treatment recommendation. Nevertheless, the current GID diagnostic criteria are biased to favor punitive gender-conversion "therapies." For example, gender-variant youth, adolescents or adults who have been shamed into the closet, forced into concealing their inner gender identities, no longer meet the diagnostic criteria of Gender Identity Disorder and are emancipated from a label of mental illness. The closet is the only exit from diagnosis.

6. **Misleading title of "Gender Identity Disorder," suggesting that gender identity is itself disordered or deficient.**

The name, Gender Identity Disorder, implies "disordered" gender identity -- that the inner identities of gender-variant individuals are not legitimate but represent perversion, delusion or immature development. In other words, the current GID diagnosis in the DSM-IV-TR implies that transwomen are nothing more than mentally ill or confused "men" and vice versa for transmen.[5]

7. **Maligning terminology, including "autogynephilia," which disrespects transitioned individuals with inappropriate pronouns and labels.**

Maligning language labels gender-variant people by assigned birth sex in disregard of inner gender identity. In other words, affirmed or transitioned transwomen are demeaned as "he" and transmen as "she." Maligning terms appear throughout the diagnostic criteria and supporting text of the GID diagnosis in the current DSM-IV-TR, where affirmed roles are termed "other sex," transsexual women are called "males" and "he," and transsexual men as "females."

Such demeaning language denies our social legitimacy and empowers defamatory social stereotypes like "a man in a dress," in the press, the courts, our workplace and our families.

8. **False positive diagnosis of those who are no longer gender dysphoric after transition and of gender nonconforming children who were never gender dysphoric.**

There is no exit clause in the diagnostic criteria for individuals whose gender dysphoria has been relieved by transition, hormones or surgical treatments, regardless of how happy or well adjusted they may be. The diagnosis is described "to have a chronic course" for adults, despite transition status or absence of distress. Children may be diagnosed with Gender Identity Disorder, solely on the basis of gender role nonconformity, without evidence of gender dysphoria. Criterion A requires only four of five listed attributes, and four of those describe violation of gender stereotypes of assigned birth sex. The fifth, describing unhappiness with birth sex, is not required to meet criterion A. Criterion B may be met by "aversion toward rough-and-tumble play and rejection of male stereotypical toys…" for natal boys and "aversion toward normative feminine clothing" for natal girls. Hence, androgynous or gender-undifferentiated children are also cast as mentally disordered.

9. **Conflation of impairment caused by prejudice with distress intrinsic to gender dysphoria.**

Criterion D of the GID diagnosis, the clinical significance criterion, was intended to require clinically significant distress or impairment to meet the accepted definition of mental disorder. Unfortunately, it fails to distinguish intrinsic distress of gender dysphoria from that caused by external societal intolerance. Lacking clarity in criterion D, external prejudice and discrimination can be misconstrued as psychological impairment for gender-variant individuals who are not distressed by physical sex characteristics or ascribed gender roles.

10. Placement in the class of sexual disorders.

In 1994, Gender Identity Disorders were moved from the class of "Disorders Usually First Evident in Infancy, Childhood or Adolescence," to the section of sexual disorders in the DSM-IV, renamed "Sexual and Gender Identity Disorders."[6] This reinforced stereotypes of sexual deviance for gender-variant people.

I hope that this list can help provide a measure of forward progress in evaluating proposals for less harmful diagnostic nomenclature in the Fifth Edition of the DSM.

[1] American Psychiatric Association, *Diagnostic and Statistical Manual of Mental Disorders*, Fourth Edition, Text Revision, Washington, D.C., 2000, pp. xxxi, xxxvii, 576-582.

[2] DSM-IV-TR Diagnostic criteria for Gender Identity Disorder of Adults and Adolescents are available online at http://www.gidreform.org/gid30285.html and for children at http://www.gidreform.org/gid3026.html .

[3] "Krishnamurti Quotes," http://www.krishnamurti.org.au/articles/krishnamurti_quotes.htm

[4] Working definition of Gender dysphoria by Dr. Randall Ehrbar and I, following our panel presentations at the 2007 convention of the American Psychological Association. It is defined in glossary of the DSM-IV-TR as "A persistent aversion toward some of all of those physical characteristics or social roles that connote one's own biological sex." (p. 823)

[5] K. Winters, "Gender Dissonance: Diagnostic Reform of Gender Identity Disorder for Adults," *Sexual and Gender Diagnoses of the Diagnostic and Statistical Manual (DSM): A Reevaluation*, Ed. Dan Karasic, MD. and Jack Drescher, MD., Haworth Press, 2005; co-published in *Journal of Psychology & Human Sexuality*, Vol. 17 issue 3, pp. 71-89, 2005.

[6] American Psychiatric Association, *Diagnostic and Statistical Manual of Mental Disorders*, Fourth Edition, 1994

A preliminary revision of this essay was posted at GID Reform Advocates: K. Winters, "Top Ten Problems with the GID Diagnosis" July 16, 2008, www.gidreform.org/blog2008Jul16.html

Epilogue:
Harm Reduction in the DSM-V

The Fifth Edition of the *Diagnostic and Statistical Manual of Mental Disorders* (DSM-V) is scheduled for publication by the American Psychiatric Association in 2012. It is the first major revision of American diagnostic nomenclature for mental disorder since 1994. Critical decisions for the organization and diagnostic criteria of the DSM-V are well underway at the time of writing. A draft of the manual is scheduled for early 2009, followed by a period of review and comment through 2010.[1, 2]

Time is of the essence for reform of gender diagnoses. In the words of the great fictional sea Captain, Jack Aubrey, "There is not a moment to lose."[3]

The DSM-V will impact the lives, civil liberties and medical care of all gender-variant people, possibly through the 2020s. The social, medical, and legal importance of the DSM is enormous, explains author Christopher Lane,

> "Not only do mental health professionals use it routinely when treating patients, but the DSM is also a bible of sorts for insurance companies deciding what disorders to

cover, as well as for clinicians, courts, prisons, pharmaceutical companies and agencies that regulate drugs."[4]

There are two prevailing views of gender diversity in American psychiatry and psychology. The emerging view is affirming and accepting, as expressed by Dr. Diane Ehrensaft on National Public Radio last May,

> "If we allow people to unfold and give them the freedom to be who they really are, we engender health. And if we try and constrict it, or bend the twig, we engender poor mental health."[5]

The traditional view is punitive, however, judging difference as disorder, something to be ashamed of - something to be "fixed." The current diagnostic categories of Gender Identity Disorder and Transvestic Fetishism in the DSM-IV-TR predominantly reflect these disparaging attitudes toward gender diversity.

The GID and TF diagnoses have long raised concern within the trans-community. Those who are distressed by their physical sex characteristics or ascribed social gender roles often need access to medically necessary transition care, and these procedures require diagnostic coding that is congruent with the treatment. At the same time, this nomenclature should respect the gender identity and expression of gender-variant children, adolescents and adults and not impose stigma of mental illness or sexual deviance on femininity, masculinity or gender diversity in themselves. As discussed in these chapters, the current GID and TF categories fail gender transcendent people in both regards.

In April 2006, the American Psychiatric Association appointed Drs. David Kupfer of the University of Pittsburgh and Darrell

Reiger, Director of the Division of Research at the APA, to head the DSM-V Task Force.[6] This was followed by announcements of 25 additional Task Force members in August 2007.[7] These included Research Director William Narrow, M.D. and Sexual and Gender Identity Disorders Work Group Chairman, Kenneth Zucker, Ph.D. of the Toronto Centre for Addiction and Mental Health (CAMH, formerly the Clarke Institute of Psychiatry).

Further work group and subcommittee appointments to the DSM-V Task Force were announced in May, 2008.[8] Peggy Cohen-Kettenis, Ph.D., of VU University in the Netherlands, was named Chair of the Gender Identity Disorders Subcommittee, and Ray Blanchard, Ph.D., of CAMH was chosen to chair the Paraphilias Subcommittee (which includes the Transvestic Fetishism diagnosis). Subsequent additions to the Sexual and GID Work Group were not announced on the APA web site until November, 2008.[9]

In 2008, gender transcendent people and allies expressed growing concern that the Sexual and GID Work Group was not sufficiently representative of clinicians and researchers with respectful views of gender diversity and transitioned individuals. The appointments of Drs. Zucker and Blanchard to leadership positions on the DSM-V sparked historically unprecedented controversy, due to their respective positions on gender-reparative therapies and paraphiliac stereotyping.[10,11] As members of the earlier DSM-IV Subcommittee on Gender Identity Disorders, Zucker and Blanchard were key to drafting the current gender diagnoses.

A collaboration of Professionals Concerned with Gender Diagnoses in the DSM advocated more balanced views in the Work Group for Sexual and Gender Identity Disorders and suggested additional members with affirming attitudes toward

171

gender diversity and social and medical transition. Organizer Arlene Lev, an author and Professor of Social Work, explained, "Addressing the complex issues we are faced with ... requires a balanced committee that represents the many perspectives and voices emanating at this seminal moment in history,"[12]

At the time of writing, the DSM-V Task Force has not responded to these requests.

In my view, the diagnosis of Transvestic Fetishism among sexual paraphilias in the DSM presents far simpler issues than GID, which carries concurrent issues about access to medical transition care. I am concerned that TF paints a broad spectrum of male-born cross-dressers, gender non-conforming individuals, and many transsexual women with stigma of mental illness and sexual perversion. I urge the DSM-V Task Force to remove the diagnostic classification of Transvestic Fetishism and related terminology of "autogynephilia" from the DSM-V.

In the 2000s, a number of proposals have emerged for reform and rethinking of the current GID diagnosis to reduce the harm of social stigma and false-positive diagnosis and also to resolve the contradiction between the current diagnostic criteria and social and medical transition. For example, in 2003, therapist Reid Vanderburgh proposed Gender Dissonance to describe a new paradigm for conceptualizing the distress of incongruence between one's experience gender identity and physical sex. He used the term in the context of identity emergence rather than diagnostic nomenclature.[13,14]

In 2003, Arlene Lev and I coauthored a presentation to the Annual Meeting of the American Psychiatric Association recommending strategies for GID reform. We suggested a replacement for GID, using Vanderburgh's term Gender

Dissonance, based on a model of distress rather than nonconformity to stereotypes of assigned birth sex.[15]

That same year, the U.K. Gender Identity Research and Education Society (GIRES) coined Atypical Gender Development to describe phenomena of diverse gender identities and expressions.[16]

In 2005, Dr. Anne Vitale presented to the Harry Benjamin International Gender Dysphoria Association (known today as the World Professional Association for Transgender Health, or WPATH) her proposal for Gender Expression Deprivation Anxiety Disorder (GEDAD) to replace Gender Identity Disorder in the DSM-V. She emphasized moving the diagnosis from the Sexual Disorders section of the DSM and moving the locus of clinical attention away from the sexological.[17,18]

Dr. Charles Moser, of the San Francisco Institute for the Advanced Study of Human Sexuality, proposed in 2008 that GID be replaced with a diagnosis termed Gender Dysphoria Disorder. He noted,

"Gender Identity Disorder is a misnomer. The 'afflicted' individuals often have no doubt about their gender identity; it just does not match their genitalia or societal expectations. The real problem is gender dysphoria, the discomfort with one's assigned gender or the profound feeling that one is the wrong gender."

His model relied on "persistent and profound discomfort with the individual's assigned gender" and clinically significant distress or impairment. Moser rejected nonconformity in gender expression as symptomatic, stating that,

"Gender variance is not a sign of mental disorder."[19]

In developing new nomenclature to replace Gender Identity Disorder, titles are especially difficult. Just as the label of GID implies that gender-variant identities are "disordered," alternative titles that lack sufficient clarity or have negative historical contexts can be controversial as well. In 2008, Mara Drummond, of the GLBT Community Center of Baltimore, proposed Incongruent Gender Dysphoria as a title for a replacement diagnostic category.[20] With the noun, *dysphoria* (from a Greek root for distress), modified by *gender* and *incongruence*, there is clearer diagnostic focus on distress rather than difference or nonconformity. Similar combinations of *gender*, *dissonance* and *dysphoria* have also been suggested.[21]

In the previous chapter, I noted ten specific issues with the title, diagnostic criteria, supporting text and placement of the current GID diagnosis in the DSM-IV-TR:

Ten Specific Issues with the GID Diagnosis	
1	Lacks clarity on debilitating distress of gender dysphoria
2	Stigma of pathology for ordinary emotions and expressions
3	Focus of pathology on nonconformity to assigned birth sex
4	Contradicts transition and hormonal and surgical treatment
5	Encourages gender-conversion therapies
6	Misleading title of "Gender Identity Disorder"
7	Maligning terms with inappropriate pronouns and labels.
8	False positive diagnosis
9	Conflation of societal prejudice with distress and impairment
10	Placement in the class of sexual disorders

I suggest that this list serve as a metric for discussing alternatives to replace Gender Identity Disorder in the DSM-V. For example, some community advocates have long called for outright elimination of GID and all diagnostic nomenclature related to gender variance. While this might address a majority of the issues listed here, I am concerned that removing all diagnostic coding that is currently used to facilitate partial access to hormonal and surgical transition care would worsen Issue #1 and fail to improve Issue #4. Thus, it would improve some concerns for some people at the expense of more harm to others. This is why I have advocated reform of the GID diagnosis, rather than removal of all diagnostic nomenclature. My personal value for GID reform is that proposed diagnostic nomenclature should lend forward-progress to as many of these issues as possible for as many people as possible.

Ultimately, replacing psychiatric diagnosis altogether with nomenclature of a physical medical condition has long been the goal of many trans-advocates concerned about twin issues of stigma and access to transition procedures. Speaking as a clinician specialized in sexual and gender issues, Arlene Lev noted that,

> "Approval for treatment should not depend on being mentally ill, but on being mentally sound enough to make empowered and healthy decisions for regarding one's body and life."[22]

To cite just a few examples, Kerry Lobel of the National Gay and Lesbian Task Force stated in 1996 that, "Reform means another diagnosis -- possibly medical -- that does not pathologize transgender people or gender-variant youth and children;"[23] and author Riki Wilchins, founder of GenderPAC, spoke of replacement by a "a non-stigmatizing physical medical condition."[24] Internist Dr. Joy Shaffer lamented in 1997 that

"Transsexualism itself does not exist as a defined entity in medical textbooks or medical school curricula."[25] At the 2007 WPATH Symposium, psychotherapist Moonhawk River Stone proposed that a medical replacement for GID, entitled Atypical Gender Identity Syndrome, be classified as an endocrine condition.[26]

Migrating the diagnosis of clinically significant gender dysphoria from mental to medical nomenclature will require education and consensus building within medical specialties and development of diagnostic criteria for physical medical categories of the *International Statistical Classification of Diseases and Related Health Problems* (ICD).[27] (The ICD contains psychiatric diagnoses as well as somatic categories, and the current psychiatric gender diagnoses in the ICD share the same shortcomings as those in the DSM.) It is also important that a medical diagnostic replacement for GID be defined in a way that does not imply disorder for trans-people who do not experience anatomic or physical dysphoria or need transition procedures.[28-29] Despite the challenges, replacing psychiatric with medical diagnostic nomenclature for gender dysphoric transsexual individuals who need access to hormonal or surgical trasition care may well be one of the most advantageous long-term strategies.

In the short term, however, I feel there is great urgency in simultaneously reducing the harm inflicted by the GID diagnosis in the DSM-V, currently under development. In my view, efforts for incremental reform of Gender Identity Disorder in the DSM are complementary to those to develop physical medical alternatives, as the next opportunity to revise the *Diagnostic and Statistical Manual of Mental Disorders* may be decades away.

As the DSM-V is drafted in the coming months, I urge all gender transcendent people to come together in solidarity and mutual support across the diversity that exists within our numbers. I request that leaders and policy advocates of the broader gay, lesbian, bisexual, transgender, intersex and queer communities lend much greater urgency to these psychiatric policy issues that impact all who vary from binary gender stereotypes. I ask psychiatric policy makers within the APA DSM-V Task Force to rethink and reform gender diagnoses to respect the human dignity, social legitimacy, and health care needs of those who transcend the bounds of our assigned birth sex.

Finally, I ask the elected leadership and Board of Trustees of the American Psychiatric Association to affirm in a public statement that gender identity and expression which differ from assigned birth sex do not, in themselves, constitute mental disorder and imply no impairment in judgment or competence. I also ask the APA to follow the example of the American Medical Association with a statement clarifying the medical necessity of hormonal and surgical transition treatments for those who suffer gender dysphoria, that is painful distress with their physical sex characteristics or ascribed gender role.

Because difference is not disease.
Because nonconformity is not pathology.
Because uniqueness is not illness[30]

[1] R. Peele, "History and Impact of APA's Leadership in Psychiatric Diagnosing," May 2008. http://www.rogerpeele.com/clinical_topics/history_of_the_dsm.asp

[2] K. Winters, "DSM 5th Edition: Status and Issues," 2008. http://www.gidreform.org/dsm5.html

[3] P. O'Brian, *Master and Commander*, Norton, 1990, p. 352

[4] C. Lane, "Opinion: Wrangling over Psychiatry's Bible," Los Angeles Times, November 16, 2008, http://www.latimes.com/news/opinion/commentary/la-oe-lane16-2008nov16,0,5678764.story

[5] A. Spiegel, "Two Families Grapple with Sons' Gender Preferences: Psychologists Take Radically Different Approaches in Therapy," National Public Radio, *All Things Considered*, May 7, 2008, http://www.npr.org/templates/story/story.php?storyId=90247842

[6] American Psychiatric Association, "APA Appoints David J. Kupfer, M.D., and Darrel A. Regier, M.D., M.P.H. To Head DSM-5 Task Force," April 2006, http://www.psych.org/MainMenu/Newsroom/NewsReleases/2006NewsReleases/06-23dsmrelease.aspx

[7] J. Yan, "APA Announces DSM-V Task Force Members," *Psychiatric News*, v. 42 n. 16, August 17, 2007, p. 10, http://pn.psychiatryonline.org/cgi/content/full/42/16/10

[8] American Psychiatric Association, "APA Names DSM-V Work Group Members: Experts to Revise Manual for Diagnosis of Mental Disorders," News Release, May 1, 2008, http://www.psych.org/MainMenu/Newsroom/NewsReleases/2008NewsReleases/dsmwg.aspx

[9] American Psychiatric Association, "Sexual and Gender Identity Disorders Work Group," http://www.psych.org/MainMenu/Research/DSMIV/DSMV/WorkGroups/SexualGID.aspx

[10] Z. Szymanski, "DSM controversy could overshadow opportunities," *Bay Area Reporter*, May 29, 2008.

http://www.ebar.com/news/article.php?sec=news&article=3018

[11] "Objection to DSM-V Committee Members on Gender Identity Disorders," Online petition, http://www.thepetitionsite.com/2/objection-to-dsm-v-committee-members-on-gender-identity-disorders

[12] A. Lev, "Sample Letters to the DSM-V Task Force of the American Psychiatric Association," Professionals Concerned with Gender Diagnoses in the DSM, http://professionals.gidreform.org/samples.html

[13] Vanderburgh R. (2001). "Gender Dissonance: A New Paradigm." Thesis for MA in Counseling Psychology (Transpersonal Psychology), Graduate School for Holistic Studies, John F. Kennedy University, Orinda, CA. [Online] See also www.transtherapist.com

[14] The term, Gender Dissonance, has previously been used in a similar context of gender dysphoria, or distress with physical sex characteristics or ascribed gender role, by authors including Jamison Green (personal correspondence, 2008) and A. Eyler and K. Wright, "Gender Identification and Sexual Orientation Among Genetic Females with Gender -Blended Self-Perception in Childhood and Adolescence," *International Journal of Transgenderism*, v. 1 n. 1, July 1997, http://www.symposion.com/ijt/ijtc0102.htm. Gender Dissonance has also been used to describe mere nonconformity of gender expression for gay and lesbian identified people. For example, see P. Doan and H. Higgins, "Cognitive Dimensions of Queer Space: The Implications of Gender Dissonance for Wayfinding in Gay and Lesbian Neighborhoods," http://www.coss.fsu.edu/durp/sites/coss.fsu.edu.durp/files/WPS_06_02_Doan.pdf

[15] K. Winters and A. Lev, "Disordering Gender Identity: Issues of Diagnostic Reform," Annual Meeting of the American Psychiatric Association, Session S24. Sexual and Gender Identity Disorders: Questions for DSM-V, San Francisco, May 19, 2003;
See also: K. Winters, "Gender Dissonance: Diagnostic Reform of Gender Identity Disorder for Adults," *Sexual and Gender Diagnoses of the Diagnostic and Statistical Manual (DSM): A Reevaluation*, Ed. Dan Karasic, MD. and Jack Drescher, MD., Haworth Press, 2005; co-published in *Journal of Psychology & Human Sexuality*, Vol. 17 issue 3, pp. 71-89, 2005.

[16] Gender Identity Research and Education Society (GIRES), "Atypical Gender Development – A Review," http://gires.org.uk/assets/atypical-gender-development.pdf

[17] Vitale, A. (2001) "Implications of Being Gender Dysphoric: A Developmental Review," *Gender and Psychoanalysis An Interdisciplinary Journal*, Vol 6 No. 2 121-141 See excerpt at http://www.avitale.com/developmentalreview.htm

[18] A. Vitale, "Notes on Gender Role Transition: Rethinking the Gender Identity Disorder Terminology in the Diagnostic and Statistical Manual of Mental Disorders IV," Harry Benjamin International Gender Dysphoria Association Conference, Bologna, Italy, April 2005. http://www.avitale.com/hbigdatalkplus2005.htm

[19] C. Moser, "Op-Ed: The DSM-V and the Gender Diagnoses," Society for Sex Therapy and Research Newsletter, v. 25 n. 2, July 2008, pp. 4-5. http://www.sstarnet.org/download/News2008Jul.pdf

[20] M. Drummond, Statement on GID reform, GID Reform Advocates, http://www.gidreform.org/advocate.html#drummond

[21] K. Winters, "Harm Reduction for Gender Disorders in the DSM-V," Philadelphia Trans Health Conference, Philadelphia PA, June 2008.

[22] A. Lev, *Transgender Emergence, Therapeutic Guidelines for Working with Gender-Variant People and Their Families*, Haworth Press, 2004, p. 181.

[23] K. Lobel, National Gay and Lesbian Task Force, "Statement of Gender Identity Disorder and Transgender People," December 1996, http://www.gendertalk.com/articles/archive/ngltf1.htm

[24] R. Wilchins, GID Reform Advocates, http://www.gidreform.org/organizations.html

[25] J. Shaffer, Foreword to G. Isreal and D. Tarver, *Transgender Care: Recommended Guidelines, Practical Information and Personal Accounts*, Temple, 1997, p.xii.

[26] M. Stone, "Shifting Paradigms: Making the Case for Moving Gender Identity Disorder Out of the Diagnostic and Statistical Manual (DSM)," World

Professional Association for Transgender Health, 20th Biennial Symposium, Chicago IL, September 2007.

[27] *International Statistical Classification of Diseases and Related Health Problems* (ICD), Version 10, 2007, http://www.who.int/classifications/apps/icd/icd10online/?gf64.htm+f64

[28] J. Cromwell, "Transmen and FTMs: Identities, bodies, genders and sexualities, University of Illinois Press, 1999, p. 121.

[29] Lev, 2004, p. 181.

[30] K. Winters, GID Reform Advocates, http://gidreform.org/

Epilogue

Appendices

Appendices

184

A: Diagnostic Criteria for Gender Identity Disorder

For adults or adolescents – code 302.85[1]

A. A strong and persistent cross-gender identification (not merely a desire for any perceived cultural advantages of being the other sex). In adolescents and adults, the disturbance is manifested by symptoms such as a stated desire to be the other sex, frequent passing as the other sex, desire to live or be treated as the other sex, or the conviction that he or she has the typical feelings and reactions of the other sex.

B. Persistent discomfort with his or her sex or sense of inappropriateness in the gender role of that sex. In adolescents and adults, the disturbance is manifested by symptoms such as preoccupation with getting rid of primary and secondary sex characteristics (e.g., request for hormones, surgery, or other procedures to physically alter sexual characteristics to simulate the other sex) or belief that he or she was born the wrong sex.

C. The disturbance is not concurrent with a physical intersex condition.

D. The disturbance causes clinically significant distress or impairment in social, occupational, or other important areas of functioning.

Specify if (for sexually mature individuals) Sexually Attracted to Males, ... Females,... Both, ... Neither.

185

For children – code 302.6

A. In children, the disturbance is manifested by four (or more) of the following:
   1. repeatedly stated desire to be, or insistence that he or she is, the other sex
   2. in boys, preference for cross-dressing or simulating female attire; in girls, insistence on wearing only stereotypical masculine clothing
   3. strong and persistent preferences for cross-sex roles in make-believe play or persistent fantasies of being the other sex
   4. intense desire to participate in the stereotypical games and pastimes of the other sex
   5. strong preferences for playmates of the other sex
B. In children, the disturbance is manifested by any of the following:
   - in boys, assertion that his penis or testes are disgusting or will disappear or assertion that it would be better not to have a penis, or aversion toward rough-and-tumble play and rejection of male stereotypical toys, games and activities;
   - in girls, rejection of urinating in a sitting position, assertion that she has or will grow a penis, or assertion that she does not want to grow breasts or menstruate, or marked aversion toward normative feminine clothing.
C. The disturbance is not concurrent with a physical intersex condition.
D. The disturbance causes clinically significant distress or impairment in social, occupational, or other important areas of functioning.

[1]American Psychiatric Association, *Diagnostic and Statistical Manual of Mental Disorders*, Fourth Edition, Text Revision, Washington, D.C., 2000, p. 581

B: Diagnostic Criteria for Transvestic Fetishism

Code 302.85[1]

A. Over a period of at least 6 months, in a heterosexual male, recurrent, intense sexually arousing fantasies, sexual urges, or behaviors involving cross-dressing.
B. The fantasies, sexual urges, or behaviors cause clinically significant distress or impairment in social, occupational, or other important areas of functioning.

Specify if: With Gender Dysphoria: if the person has persistent discomfort with gender role or identity.

[1]American Psychiatric Association, *Diagnostic and Statistical Manual of Mental Disorders*, Fourth Edition, Text Revision, Washington, D.C., 2000, p. 574

C: DSM-V Policy-Makers for Gender Diagnoses

The DSM-V is under development by a Task Force, whose highest levels were appointed by the American Psychiatric Association in September, 2007. The Work Groups and Subcommittees, responsible for individual diagnostic categories were first named on May 1st, 2008,[1] with some positions (including Pfäfflin and Kafka) added in July, 2008.

The following list includes Task Force members involved with diagnostic categories of Gender Identity Disorder and Transvestic Fetishism.[2] At this time, members of an advisory group to the Sexual and Gender Identity Disorders Work Group and a task force for treatment recommendations have not yet been named by the APA.

189

DSM-V Task Force

David J. Kupfer, M.D. (Chair)
Thomas Detre Professor and Chair
Department of Psychiatry
University of Pittsburgh School of Medicine
Medical Director and Director of Research
Western Psychiatric Institute and Clinic
Pittsburgh, PA

Darrel A. Regier, M.D., M.P.H.
(Vice Chair)
Director, Division of Research
American Psychiatric Association
Executive Director
American Psychiatric Institute for
Research and Education
Arlington, VA

William E. Narrow, M.D., M.P.H.M
Research Director
Division of Research
American Psychiatric Association
Arlington, VA

Sexual and Gender Identity Disorders Work Group

Kenneth J. Zucker, Ph.D. (Chair)
Former Member, DSM-IV Subcommittee on GID
Head, Gender Identity Service Clinic, Child,
Youth, and Family Program
Centre for Addiction and Mental Health
Toronto, Ontario, Canada

Gender Identity Disorders Subcommittee

Peggy T. Cohen-Kettenis, Ph.D. (Chair)
Professor of Medical Psychology
Head of the Department of Medical Psychology,
VU University Medical Center
Director, Gender Dysphoria Expertise Center
Amsterdam, The Netherlands

Jack Drescher, M.D.
Clinical Assistant Professor of Psychiatry,
New York Medical College
Associate Attending Psychiatrist, St. Luke's-
Roosevelt Hospital Center
New York, NY

Heino F. L. Meyer-Bahlburg, Dr. rer. nat.
Former Member, DSM-IV Subcommittee on GID
Professor of Clinical Psychology (in Psychiatry),
College of Physicians & Surgeons of
Columbia University,
Research Scientist
New York State Psychiatric Institute
New York, NY

Friedemann Pfäfflin, M.D., Ph.D.
Professor of Psychotherapy
Head of the Forensic Psychotherapy Unit
Ulm University, Germany
former President HBIGDA (WPATH)
co-founder, Intl Jour of Transgenderism

Paraphilias Subcommittee

Ray Blanchard, Ph.D. (Chair)
Former Member, DSM-IV Subcommittee on GID
Professor, Department of Psychiatry
University of Toronto
Head of Clinical Sexology Services

191

Centre for Addiction and Mental Health
Toronto, Ontario, Canada

Richard B. Krueger, M.D.
Medical Director, Sexual Behavior Clinic
New York State Psychiatric Institute,
Associate Clinical Professor of Psychiatry
Department of Psychiatry
Columbia University
New York, NY

Niklas Långström, M.D., Ph.D.
Associate Professor of Child and Adolescent
Psychiatry
Head of Centre for Violence Prevention
Karolinska Institutet
Stockholm, Sweden

Martin P. Kafka, M.D.
Associate Clinical Professor of Psychiatry
Harvard University
Clinical Associate in Psychiatry
McLean Hospital
Belmont, MA

1 American Psychiatric Association, "APA Names DSM-V Work Group Members," News Release, May 1, 2008, http://www.psych.org/MainMenu/Newsroom/NewsReleases/2008NewsReleases/dsmwg.aspx

2 American Psychiatric Association, "Sexual and Gender Identity Disorders Work Group," http://www.psych.org/MainMenu/Research/DSMIV/DSMV/WorkGroups/SexualGID.aspx

D: Labels, Titles and Terms

"Oh my!"

The following list describes the most common terms I use to discuss issues of gender diversity and mental health policy. It is not comprehensive and does not imply a consensus within the trans-community on their use —far from it.

In social movements among marginalized people, there is often tension between those who strive to assimilate with the dominant culture, to blend in, and those who strive to change the dominant culture to extend dignity and equality to all. There is often tension between those who strive to build coalition and solidarity among the oppressed versus those who separate and distance themselves from others who are even more marginalized. Out of this tension, terms and labels of human diversity become the focus of passionate controversy and are subject to change without notice.

I strive to take responsibility for my own language, clarify the meaning I ascribe to my words, and learn from the feedback I receive from others. I have found that much misunderstanding stems from ambiguity between terms of social identity, human phenomena and psychiatric diagnosis. They are very different and serve different purposes. For terms of social identity, like *transgender*, my personal value is to err on the side of inclusion rather than exclusion. I do not intend to impose unwanted social identities on others, but nor do I wish to exclude people in our community who have suffered exclusion their whole lives. For terms of human phenomena, such as *gender dysphoria*, I feel that clarity is important. For diagnostic nomenclature, such as the derogatory title of *Gender Identity Disorder*, I believe the priority should be on harm reduction – to err on the side of limiting diagnosis to only those who would clearly benefit from diagnosis and meet scientific definitions of disorder. For terms of multiple contexts, such as *transsexual* (which may describe social identity, human phenomenon or psychiatric diagnosis), it is important to specify the intended meaning.

Affirmed
{Son/Daughter/Boy/Girl/Man/Woman/Female/Male} –*social identity*. Acknowledging the gender identity of individuals (always termed with respect to the person's expressed identity, not assigned birth sex.) Preferred by TransYouth Family Allies to describe youth.[1]

Anatomic Dysphoria –*phenomenon*. One type of gender dyphoria associated with persistent distress with current or anticipated (for preadolescent youth) physical sex characteristics that are incongruent with gender identity.

Cross-Dresser –*social identity*. People who wear clothing usually assigned to the opposite sex.[2] The term or its abbreviation CD are commonly associated with heterosexual males who identity primarily as male. Women in Western cultures less commonly identify as cross-dressers, since they are afforded more freedom of gender expression than men. The clinical term of mental disorder and sexual deviance, *transvestite*, is considered pejorative by many cross-dressers, though it remains a common term of social identity in Latin cultures.

FTM/MTF – *phenomena*. Shorthand for direction of social or medical transition: female-to-male and male-to-female, respectively. Generally, FTM refers to transmen and MTF to

194

transwomen. However, these acronyms are controversial among those who feel they are too restricted to binary sex stereotypes and to some individuals, who prefer trans-to male (TtoM) and trans-to-female (TtoF). On the other hand, this TtoM/TtoF notation is rejected by those who socially identify as both trans and male (or female), post-transition. Therefore, I use MTF and FTM only in the sense of the general direction of transition from a masculine or feminine birth-assignment to a space on the sex and gender spectra that differs from birth-assignment.

Gender *—inclusive of multiple phenomena and social identities.* A very broad multidimensional term that encompasses myriad combinations of human attributes that may be masculine, feminine, both or neither. Dimensions of gender include gender identity and gender expression, which may or may not correspond to each other or to social stereotypes of birth sex.

I also prefer to include physical sex and sexual orientation, each with its own broad spectrum of diversity, as dimensions of gender. This taxonomy reflects my view that humans are more than behavioral automata and illustrates the roles of the closet and social intolerance in suppressing gender diversity. It differs from that of Butler[5] and others who consider all aspects of sex, sexuality and gender subordinate to "gender performativity," which resembles what I call gender expression.

Gender Dysphoria *—phenomenon.* Persistent distress with one's current or anticipated physical sexual characteristics or current ascribed gender role.[3] It is defined more ambiguously in the DSM-IV-TR[4] and prior editions. The term was originally proposed as diagnostic nomenclature, "gender dysphoria syndrome," by Fisk in the early 1970s.[7]

Since gender identity, arguably the most important component of gender, is not the actual subject of distress, gender dysphoria might be more accurately replaced by specific terms such as "anatomic dysphoria" and "gender role dysphoria."

Gender Expression *–phenomenon.* The external social presentation of masculinity, femininity, both or neither, which may differ from biological sex or gender assigned at birth or inner gender identity. In the case of a gender-variant person forced or shamed into the closet, gender expression may be opposite to gender identity.

Gender Identity *–phenomenon.* The internal sense of masculinity or femininity that a person experiences, not always congruent with biological sex or gender assigned at birth. Gender identity is who you are not who you like.[1]

I have observed that gender identity can be hidden or closeted but have not seen evidence that it can be coerced or changed. The adage by Virginia Prince that "Gender is between the ears,"[6] would describe what I call gender identity rather than gender.

Gender Reflex *–phenomenon.* The propensity of cultures, institutions and individuals to reduce all people to binary masculine and feminine gender stereotypes with associated presumptions of physical sex.

(Even trans-people are not immune to this habit; we just feel more guilty when we catch ourselves doing it.)

Gender Transcendence *–phenomenon.* Transcending the bounds of stereotypes associated with physical sex characteristics or assigned birth sex.

I prefer gender transcendence over transgender to describe the breadth of human gender diversity beyond binary stereotypes. See gender variance.

Gender Variance *–phenomenon.* Difference in gender identity or expression from stereotypes associated with physical sex characteristics or birth sex. Preferred by TransYouth Family Allies to describe gender diversity in children and youth for whom labels of social identity would be presumptuous.[1] See gender transcendence.

Maligning Language *–phenomenon.* Of the disrespectful language faced by gender-variant people, I feel that none is more damaging or hurtful than that which disregards our gender identities, denies affirmed social roles of those who have transitioned, and reduces us to our assigned birth sex. I am speaking of affirmed transwomen being called "he" and transmen being called "she." I use the term Maligning Language to describe this specific kind of verbal violence and believe it is respectful to address people in the sense of their identified or expressed gender, which may differ from their assigned birth sex.

Sex *–phenomenon.* Physical sex, which is comprised of a number of attributes: anatomical, physiological, hormonal, reproductive, genetic, chromosomal, brain-sex and birth-assignment. Physical sex may align with gender identity and social gender expression or may differ in myriad ways. According to the Organisation Intersexués Internationales, one in 100 people are born with bodies differing from standard male or female phenotypes or genotypes.[8]

Transgender *–social identity.* An umbrella community term describing a wide diversity of people who differ in gender identity or gender expression from social expectations of assigned birth sex. This may include those who identify as transsexual, transitioned, cross-dresser, bi or dual gender, genderqueer, gender nonconforming, and many other descriptions. Often abbreviated *Trans*, Transgender as an inclusive social identity is often conflated with *transgenderist*, a much narrower exclusive term coined by Virginia Prince in the 1970s to describe those who transition full-time in social role without a desire for surgical procedures.[9] She earlier used the term *transgenderal* in a similar context. [10] Transgender as an adjective with no suffix is commonly considered more respectful than *transgendered* or as a noun. Not all people in various categories of gender diversity socially identify as Transgender.

I prefer to use transgender in its most inclusive sense and as a term of social identity. I use gender transcendence or gender variance to describe phenomena of gender diversity.

Transsexual *–social identity.* A term describing a person whose inner gender identity is incongruent with her or his born physical sex characteristics. Many transsexual individuals seek medical treatments to bring their bodies into harmony with their gender identities, though not all are able or choose to do so. Transsexual, coined by psychiatrist Harry Benjamin in the 1960s,[11] is most respectfully used as an adjective. Although the term is often used to describe the phenomenon of sex/gender incongruence, not all people who have transitioned socially or medically identify as Transsexual. For example, Transsexualism is a label of mental disorder in the *International Statistical Classification of Diseases and Related Health Problems* (ICD)[12] and is considered pejorative by some people outside North America. Some post-operative people regard Transsexual identity as transitional and refer to it in the past tense. Some Transsexual individuals also identify with the broader transgender community; others do not.

Therefore, I prefer to use Transsexual as a term of social self-identity, which may include pre-operative, post-operative or non-operative individuals.

1 "Learning the Lingo," TransYouth Family Allies, 2008,
http://imatyfa.org/permanent_files/learning-the-lingo-06-08.pdf

2 A. Lev, A. Lev, *Transgender Emergence, Therapeutic Guidelines for Working with Gender-Variant People and Their Families*, Haworth Press, 2004, p. 396.

3 Working definition of Gender dysphoria by Dr. Randall Ehrbar and I following our panel presentations at the 2007 convention of the American Psychological Association.

4 Defined in glossary of the DSM-IV-TR as "A persistent aversion toward some of all of those physical characteristics or social roles that connote one's own biological sex." (2000, p. 823)

5 J. Butler, *Gender Trouble: Feminism and the Subversion of Identity*, Routledge, 1989.

6 V. Prince, "Sex versus Gender," Proceedings of the 2nd Interdisciplinary Symposium on Gender Dysphoria Syndrome, Stanford, Calif., 1973, pp. 20-24

7 N. Fisk, "Gender dysphoria syndrome. (The how, what, and why of a disease)," In D. Laub & P. Gandy (Eds.), *Proceedings of the second interdisciplinary symposium on gender dysphoria syndrome* , Stanford, 1973, pp. 7-14.

8 "How Common is Intersex? Prevalence of Variations," Organisation Intersexués Internationales, 2008,
http://www.intersexualite.org/how_common_is_intersex.pdf

9 V. Prince, "The 'Transcendents' or 'Trans' People," *Transvestia*, v. 16, n. 95, pp. 81-92.

10 P. Bentler and C. Prince, "Personality Characteristics of Male Transvestites III," *Journal of Abnormal Psychology*, v. 72, n. 2, pp. 140-143.

11 H. Benjamin, *The Transsexual Phenomenon*, Julian Press, 1966, p. 23.

12 *International Statistical Classification of Diseases and Related Health Problems* (ICD), Version 10, 2007,
http://www.who.int/classifications/apps/icd/icd10online/?gf64.htm+f64

Index

Bradley, 25, 27, 30, 31, 42, 103, 104, 105, 112, 124, 129, 138
Burgess, 156, 160
Burke, 106, 114, 152, 153, 159
Burns, 108
Butler, 200

C

Centre for Addiction and Mental Health, 26, 46, 55, 82, 118, 156, 190, 192
Clarke Institute of Psychiatry, 26, 46, 55, 82, 83, 118, 156
Cohen-Kettenis, 112, 171, 191
Cole, 105, 113
Conway, vii, 84, 85, 89, 94, 99, 107, 108, 113, 114, 126, 128, 139
Corporate Equality Index, 66, 68, 69
cross-dresser, 198
Cross-Dresser, 194
cross-dressing, 2, 20, 22, 33, 34, 35, 36, 37, 119, 123, 131, 138, 156, 186, 188
Cross-dressing, 34

D

Davis, 155
De Vries, 105, 112
Diagnostic and Statistical Manual of Mental Disorders, 1, 2, 5, 8, 11, 16, 17, 20, 29, 30, 33, 41, 46, 49, 58, 61, 68, 73, 77, 81, 88, 91, 96, 99, 101, 112, 117, 126, 138, 144, 146, 159, 161, 167, 169, 187, 188
Dobson, 45
Dreger, 108, 109, 115, 126, 139
Drescher, 16, 43, 58, 68, 71, 77, 112, 115, 167, 179, 191
Drummond, vii, 31, 112, 174, 180
DSM-V Task Force, 6, 25, 48, 76, 98, 144, 190

E

Ehrensaft, 103, 170
Ensler, 155, 159
equifinality, 133

F

falsifiability of hypotheses, 133
Fedoroff, 55, 58

204

V

Vitale, viii, 173, 180

W

Wålinder[13], 84
Wilchins, vii, 142, 175, 180
Winters, iii, iv, 16, 17, 29, 31, 41, 42, 43, 49, 58, 59, 68, 69, 77, 78, 89, 99, 100, 112, 113, 116, 127, 129, 138, 139, 140, 146, 147, 160, 167, 179, 207
World Professional Association for Transgender Health, 14, 17, 47, 58, 61, 65, 68, 69, 84, 113, 207

Z

Zucker, 13, 17, 24, 25, 27, 30, 31, 37, 42, 48, 49, 83, 88, 101, 102, 103, 104, 106, 109, 112, 114, 124, 129, 138, 143, 190

About the Author

Kelley Winters, Ph.D. is a proud parent, retired engineer, writer and community advocate on issues of transgender medical policy. She is the founder of GID Reform Advocates, a member of the World Professional Association for Transgender Health and an Advisory Board Member for the Matthew Shepard Foundation and TransYouth Family Allies. She has presented papers on the psychiatric classification of gender diversity at annual conventions of the American Psychiatric Association, the American Psychological Association, the American Counseling Association and the Association of Women in Psychology. Her articles have appeared in a number of mental health journals and in two books. Dr. Winters assisted in drafting the current human rights ordinances in Boulder and Denver, Colorado. She was instrumental in reform of Colorado drivers license policy in 2006 and in adding Gender Identity and Expression to employment policies of the Hewlett-Packard Company. Dr. Winters received the Colorado Pride Award in 1999 and the 2002 Sonja's Dream Lifetime Achievement Award and 2007 Melissa Chapman Award for Social Change from the Gender Identity Center of Colorado. She currently lives in Colorado and enjoys skiing, hiking and landscape photography.

Made in the USA
San Bernardino, CA
01 September 2016